Abdominal X-rays

for Medical Students

This book is dedicated to all teaching radiologists and their students.

This title is also available as an e-book.
For more details, please see
www.wiley.com/buy/9781118600559
or scan this QR code:

Abdominal X-rays
for Medical Students

Christopher G.D. Clarke, MBChB
Radiology Registrar and Honorary Lecturer in Human Anatomy
Nottingham University Hospitals
Nottingham, UK

Anthony E.W. Dux, MB BS, FRCR
Former Consultant Radiologist and Honorary Senior Lecturer
University Hospitals of Leicester
Leicester, UK

WILEY Blackwell

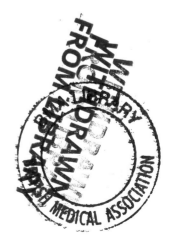

This edition first published 2015 © 2015 by John Wiley & Sons, Ltd.

Registered Office
John Wiley & Sons, Ltd., The Atrium, Southern Gate, Chichester, West Sussex, PO19 8SQ, UK

Editorial Offices
9600 Garsington Road, Oxford, OX4 2DQ, UK
The Atrium, Southern Gate, Chichester, West Sussex, PO19 8SQ, UK
350 Main Street, Malden, MA 02148-5020, USA

For details of our global editorial offices, for customer services and for information about how to apply for permission to reuse the copyright material in this book please see our website at www.wiley.com/wiley-blackwell

Library of Congress Cataloging-in-Publication Data

Clarke, Christopher, 1986– , author.
   Abdominal X-rays for medical students / Christopher G.D. Clarke, Anthony E.W. Dux.
      p. ;   cm.
   Includes bibliographical references and index.
   ISBN 978-1-118-60055-9 (pbk.)
I. Dux, Anthony, author.   II. Title.
[DNLM: 1. Radiography, Abdominal–methods–Atlases.   2. Abdomen–pathology–Atlases.
3. Digestive System Diseases–radiography–Atlases. WI 17]
   RC944
   617.5′507572–dc23

                              2014047517

A catalogue record for this book is available from the British Library.

Wiley also publishes its books in a variety of electronic formats. Some content that appears in print may not be available in electronic books.

Cover images: Radiographs showing calcification in the wall of the abdominal aorta; fetus in situ; dilated small bowel; gas-filled distended stomach; toxic megacolon; various ingested foreign objects. Illustrations by Christopher Clarke.

Set in 10/13pt Frutiger by SPi Publisher Services, Pondicherry, India
Printed and bound in Singapore by Markono Print Media Pte Ltd

1   2015

Contents

Preface

The abdominal radiograph is commonly encountered within the hospital setting, and often junior doctors are the first to review and act upon the radiograph findings. Medical students therefore need to learn how to interpret basic signs and pathology on an abdominal radiograph.

This book is a follow-up to *Chest X-rays for Medical Students*, which Anthony and I wrote a few years ago to help medical students with chest radiographs. Since publishing the chest X-ray book, I have entered clinical radiology training at Nottingham University Hospitals NHS Trust and passed fellowship exams. Anthony has retired, returning a few days a week to continue reporting and teaching. This book has taken approximately 12 months to write and much longer to collect all the radiographs featured within.

The most novel and exciting aspect of *Abdominal X-rays for Medical Students* is the way colour overlays are used to highlight the anatomy and pathology. This way of 'marking' the radiographs separates this book from others and makes it easy to appreciate the sign or pathology of interest. Generally, two radiographs are displayed side by side with the radiograph on the right marked out in colour and the radiograph on the left unmarked for comparison. This makes it easy to compare and identify the abnormality on the unmarked radiograph. Some signs and pathologies are difficult to appreciate, and I experimented with different enhancement techniques until I found one that worked. The result of this was that I have ended up using a range of different techniques to show or enhance pathology in this book.

This book is not intended to be used as an encyclopaedic reference but as a colourful and informative teaching aid to help medical students, junior doctors, radiographers and nurses learn the basics of abdominal X-ray interpretation in a simplified, logical and systematic way. We try to avoid confusing terms and fully explain any commonly used radiographic signs such as *thumbprinting* or *Rigler's sign*.

I hope that by the end of this book, you should have a system to use for analysing and presenting abdominal radiographs and know how to recognise the important common pathologies on an abdominal X-ray.

We are constantly improving and refining this teaching resource for future students, so would really appreciate any feedback or suggestions you may have. Please feel free to contact us with any ideas you have.

I hope that you enjoy using this book.

Christopher G.D. Clarke

Acknowledgements

First, we would like to thank the staff at Nottingham University Hospitals NHS Trust, University Hospitals of Leicester NHS Trust and Derby Hospitals NHS Foundation Trust, without whose dedication and work none of this would be possible. We would like to acknowledge our colleagues who have read this workbook and made numerous suggestions and contributions including many of the Nottingham and Leicester clinical radiology trainees. It would be impossible to name everyone, but we are very grateful.

We would like to thank Dr Tim Taylor and Benjamin Troth for providing many excellent radiograph examples. A special thanks goes to Dr Gill Turner for providing us with access to her fantastic collection of abdominal radiographs, many of which are used in this book. I just hope the colouring has done her collection justice!

Special thanks also go to the many medical students who attended focus groups, lectures and teaching sessions and gave fantastic feedback. I would like to thank Elizabeth Bridges, Sally Wege, Stephanie Ainley and Mark Evans for giving up their time to help in the very early stages of writing. Also I would like to thank Theodora Goodwin, Sian Dobbs, Charlotte Bee, Gemma Dracup and Jenna Harris for their feedback on the draft. Their suggestions and contributions shaped this book and were invaluable. We are grateful to Carole and David Clarke and Gill Turner for taking time to proof read the draft and provide numerous suggestions to improve the book. Thank you to William Clarke and George Booth for their help with the diagrams and photos.

The 'Polo' name and image is reproduced with the kind permission of Société des Produits Nestlé S.A.

Thanks to Martin Davies and Karen Moore from Wiley-Blackwell for their patience and for giving us the opportunity to see our work published again. To all our friends that have supported us and to all those people who remain unnamed in this acknowledgement, we are very grateful.

Finally, thank you to Stewart Petersen for his advice, encouragement and support in publishing *Chest X-rays for Medical Students*. Without his contribution and kindness, *Abdominal X-rays for Medical Students* would never have been developed.

Learning objectives checklist

(Keep track of your learning by ticking the ☐ when you have covered that topic)

By the end of this workbook, students should:

- Have a basic understanding of what X-rays are and how the image is produced. ☐
- Have a system for analysing (ABCDE) and presenting an abdominal radiograph. ☐
- Know how to recognise the following on a plain abdominal radiograph:
  - Pneumoperitoneum (gas in the peritoneal cavity) ☐
  - Pneumoretroperitoneum (gas in the retroperitoneal space) ☐
  - Pneumobilia (gas in the biliary tree) ☐
  - Portal venous gas (gas in the portal vein) ☐
  - Dilated small bowel ☐
  - Dilated large bowel ☐
  - Volvulus ☐
  - Dilated stomach ☐
  - Hernia ☐
  - Bowel wall inflammation ☐
  - Faecal loading ☐
  - Faecal impaction ☐
  - Gallstones in the gallbladder (cholelithiasis) ☐
  - Renal stones (urolithiasis) ☐
  - Bladder stones ☐
  - Nephrocalcinosis ☐
  - Pancreatic calcification ☐
  - Adrenal calcification ☐
  - Abdominal aortic aneurysm (AAA) calcification ☐
  - Fetus ☐
  - Calcified costal cartilage ☐
  - Phleboliths ('vein stones') ☐
  - Calcified mesenteric lymph nodes ☐
  - Calcified uterine fibroids ☐
  - Prostate calcification ☐
  - Abdominal aortic calcification (normal calibre) ☐
  - Splenic artery calcification ☐
  - Pelvic fractures – 3 Polo rings test ☐
  - Sclerotic and lucent bone lesions ☐
  - Spine pathology ☐
  - Solid organ enlargement ☐
  - Surgical clips/staples/sutures ☐
  - Urinary catheter ☐
  - Supra-pubic catheter ☐
  - Nasogastric (NG) and nasojejunal (NJ) tubes ☐
  - Flatus tube ☐
  - Surgical drain ☐
  - Nephrostomy catheter ☐
  - Peritoneal dialysis (PD) catheter ☐
  - Gastric band device ☐
  - Percutaneous endoscopic gastrostomy (PEG)/radiologically inserted gastrostomy (RIG) ☐
  - Stoma bag ☐
  - Stents ☐
  - Inferior vena cava (IVC) filter ☐
  - Intra-uterine device (IUD) ☐
  - Pessary ☐
  - Retained surgical swab ☐
  - Swallowed objects ☐
  - Objects inserted per-rectum (PR) ☐
  - Clothing artefact ☐
  - Piercings ☐
  - Body packer ☐
  - Lung bases ☐

About X-rays

What are X-rays?

X-rays are a form of **ionising radiation**. They are part of the electromagnetic spectrum and have sufficient energy to cause ionisations. They contain more energy than ultraviolet (UV) waves but less energy than gamma rays.

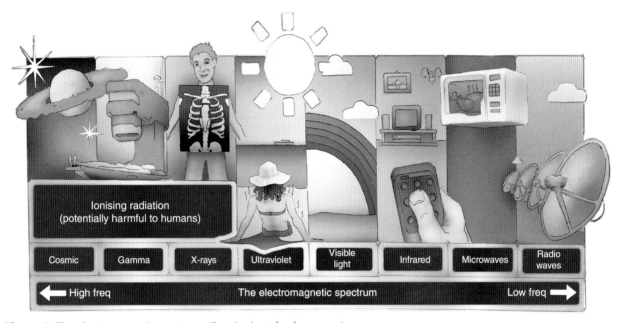

Figure 1: The electromagnetic spectrum (Freq is short for frequency).

Radiation is the transfer of energy in the form of particles or waves.

Ionising radiation is the radiation with sufficient energy to cause ionisations, which is a process whereby radiation removes an outer shell electron from an atom. Thus ionising radiation is able to cause changes on a molecular level in biologically important molecules (e.g. DNA).

Uses of ionising radiation include conventional X-rays (plain radiographs), contrast studies, computed tomography (CT), nuclear medicine and positron emission tomography (PET).

How are X-rays produced?

X-rays are produced by focusing a high-energy beam of electrons onto a metal target (e.g. tungsten). The electrons hit the metal target and some will have enough energy to knock out another electron from the inner shell of one of the metal atoms. As a result, electrons from higher energy levels then fill up this vacancy and

Abdominal X-rays for Medical Students, First Edition. Christopher G.D. Clarke and Anthony E.W. Dux.
© 2015 John Wiley & Sons, Ltd. Published 2015 by John Wiley & Sons, Ltd.

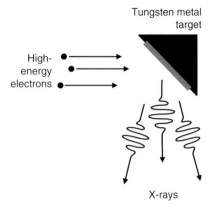

Tungsten metal target

High-energy electrons

X-rays

Figure 2: X-ray production.

X-rays are emitted in the process. Producing X-rays this way is extremely inefficient (~0.1%), so most of the energy is wasted as heat. This is why X-ray tubes need to have advanced cooling mechanisms. The X-rays produced then pass through the patient and onto a detector mechanism which produces an image.

How do X-rays make an image?

Main points include the following:

1. The resulting image on the X-ray detector is a **two-dimensional (2D) representation of a three-dimensional (3D) structure**.
2. While passing through a patient the X-ray beam is absorbed in proportion to the cube of the atomic number of the various tissues through which it passes. By convention, the greater the amount of radiation hitting a detector, the darker the image will be. Therefore, the less "dense" a material is, the more X-rays get through and the darker the image. Conversely the more "dense" a material is, the more X-rays are absorbed and the image appears whiter. Materials of low "density" appear darker than those of high "density".
3. **Structures can only be seen if there is sufficient contrast with surrounding tissues** (contrast is the difference in absorption between one tissue and another).

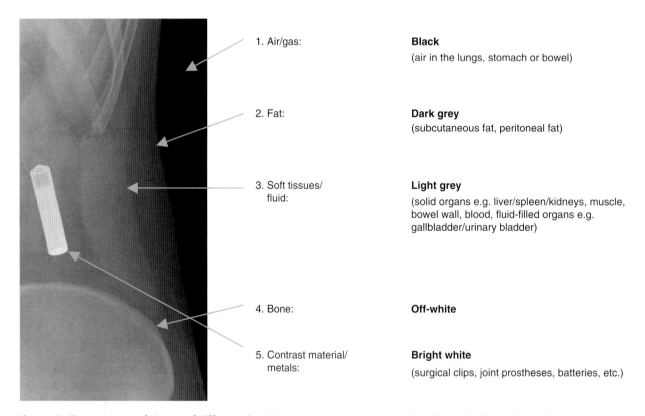

1. Air/gas: **Black**
(air in the lungs, stomach or bowel)

2. Fat: **Dark grey**
(subcutaneous fat, peritoneal fat)

3. Soft tissues/ fluid: **Light grey**
(solid organs e.g. liver/spleen/kidneys, muscle, bowel wall, blood, fluid-filled organs e.g. gallbladder/urinary bladder)

4. Bone: **Off-white**

5. Contrast material/ metals: **Bright white**
(surgical clips, joint prostheses, batteries, etc.)

Figure 3: The spectrum of tissues of different densities as seen on a conventional radiograph. The radiograph example shows the left lumbar region of a patient who swallowed a battery.

How are X-ray images (radiographs) stored?

In some hospitals radiographs are printed onto X-ray film, but most places now use a computer-based digital radiograph storage system for storing X-ray images, thereby eliminating the need for film.

This system is known as **P**icture **A**rchiving and **C**ommunication **S**ystem (**PACS**). Doctors and other healthcare professionals are able to view the images (radiographs) on a computer screen, making it easy to manipulate the image (e.g. changing the contrast, zooming in/out, etc).

The advantages are ease of access, both locally and internationally, cost saving and no more lost films. The disadvantages are the initial cost and the risk of a system failure, which could be potentially catastrophic.

Radiation hazards

Radiation hazards occur as a result of damage to cells by radiation. Actively dividing cells are particularly sensitive (e.g. bone marrow, lymph glands and gonads). Damage takes many forms including cell death, mitotic inhibition and chromosome/genetic damage leading to mutations.

The radiation dose from an abdominal X-ray is approximately 30 times more than that of a chest X-ray and equivalent to 2 months of background radiation. It is therefore important to optimise the radiation dose to as low as reasonably achievable, while still obtaining an image of good diagnostic quality. The safety of patients and the use of ionising radiation for medical exposures are subject to specific legislation in the UK – the Ionising Radiation (Medical Exposure) Regulations or IRMER.

The Ionising Radiation (Medical Exposure) Regulations

Introduced in 2000, with a few subsequent amendments since, it lays down the basic measures for radiation protection for patients. It refers to three main people involved in protecting the patient:
1. The **Referrer** (a doctor or other accredited health professional [e.g. emergency nurse practitioner] requesting the exposure)
   - Must provide adequate and relevant clinical information to enable the practitioner to justify the exposure
2. The **Practitioner** (usually a radiologist, who justifies the exposure)
   - Decides on the appropriate imaging and justifies any exposure to radiation on a case-by-case basis.
   - **Potential benefit must outweigh the risk to the patient** (*e.g. a CT head scan on a 1-year-old adds a 1/500 lifetime risk of cancer and increases the risk of cataract formation. The benefit of this scan must therefore outweigh these risks to the child.*)
3. The **Operator** (usually a radiographer, who performs practical aspects)
   - Ensures that the above two stages have been completed appropriately
   - Keeps all justifiable exposure as low as reasonably possible by
     i. minimising the number of X-ray radiographs taken
     ii. focusing the X-ray beam to the area of interest
     iii. keeping exposure as low as reasonably achievable

In women of reproductive age

- Minimise radiation exposure of abdomen and pelvis.
- Ask women of reproductive age if they could be pregnant, and avoid radiation exposure to them. The most critical periods are during the first and second trimester. From the standpoint of future development, the foetus is considered to be most radiosensitive during the second trimester when foetal organogenesis is taking place. X-rays of the abdomen and pelvis should be delayed, if possible, to a time when foetal sensitivity is reduced (i.e. post 24 weeks' gestation, or ideally until the baby is born).
- Exposure to remote areas (chest, skull and limbs) may be undertaken with minimal foetal exposure at any time during pregnancy.

Indications for an abdominal X-ray

Only request an abdominal X-ray if it is the most appropriate test to answer the clinical question. Indications for a plain abdominal X-ray are as follows:

- **Suspected bowel obstruction**
  To look for dilated loops of small or large bowel or a dilated stomach.
- **Suspected perforation**
  To look for evidence of pneumoperitoneum. An **erect chest X-ray** should always be requested at the same time to look for free gas under the diaphragm.
- **Moderate-to-severe undifferentiated abdominal pain**
  May be useful if the provisional diagnosis includes any of the following: toxic megacolon, bowel obstruction and perforation.
- **Suspected foreign body**
  To look for the presence of radiopaque foreign bodies.
- **Renal tract calculi follow-up**
  To look for the presence or movement of known renal tract calculi.

For most other clinical situations, an **abdominal X-ray is not recommended** as there is a more appropriate alternative test. Common examples include:

- *Abdominal trauma:* A CT scan of the abdomen and pelvis with intravenous contrast is much more sensitive and specific at looking for evidence of solid organ, bowel or bony injury and may identify the site of significant active bleeding.
- *Right upper quadrant abdominal pain:* An ultrasound scan of the abdomen is recommended to look for evidence of gallstones, inflamed gallbladder or an obstructed common bile duct.
- *Suspected intra-abdominal collection:* A CT scan of the abdomen and pelvis is recommended to look for a source of infection (collection of pus or fluid).
- *Acute upper gastrointestinal bleeding:* Endoscopy is indicated and enables diagnosis in most cases and can be used to deliver haemostatic therapy. If initial endoscopy is negative, then angiography or CT angiography may be useful to identify the source of the bleeding.
- *Suspected intra-abdominal malignancy:* A CT scan of the abdomen and pelvis is recommended to look for a malignancy and can be used to help stage the malignancy if found.
- *Constipation:* This is usually a clinical diagnosis without the need for any imaging tests. There is no evidence correlating abdominal X-ray findings with constipation. The only exception is in elderly patients where an abdominal X-ray may be useful to show the extent of faecal impaction, but does not diagnose constipation.

Abdominal X-rays for Medical Students, First Edition. Christopher G.D. Clarke and Anthony E.W. Dux.
© 2015 John Wiley & Sons, Ltd. Published 2015 by John Wiley & Sons, Ltd.

Abdominal X-ray views

The standard view is an **anterior–posterior (AP) supine abdominal X-ray (AXR)**. Almost all AXRs are taken AP supine. In general, you should assume that an abdominal radiograph is taken AP supine unless otherwise stated.

AP Supine abdominal X-ray

The patient lies supine (on their back). The X-ray tube is positioned overhead in front of the patient, so the X-rays pass in the AP direction. The patient is asked to hold their breath (so that breathing movement will not make the image blurry) and the X-ray is taken.

The abdominal radiographs are performed in the supine position as it is generally easier for patients to lie on their back, especially if they are unwell or post-operative.

The average detector used to image the abdomen is 35 × 43 cm, which is slightly smaller than the normal average adult abdomen. This means that two or more radiographs are sometimes needed to image the entire abdomen. It is therefore important to check whether a second radiograph has been taken before reporting an abdominal X-ray.

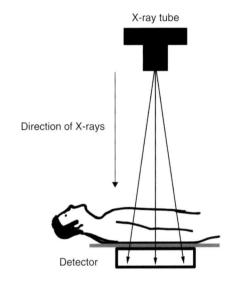

Figure 4: Anterior–posterior (AP) supine abdominal X-ray.

Other views

- **Erect AXR** (patient upright): It is very rarely performed nowadays as it has little diagnostic value when compared to a CT scan of the abdomen and pelvis. The erect AXR may demonstrate gas–fluid levels (gas rises, fluid sinks) and in the past was useful in suspected bowel obstruction.
- **Left lateral decubitus AXR** (patient lying on their left side): It is very rarely performed nowadays although is sometimes used in children to avoid high-dose CT when trying to diagnose suspected bowel perforation. The patient usually lies on their left side (as opposed to the right side) so any free intra-peritoneal gas is seen outlined against the liver edge (see Figure 28).
- **Erect chest X-ray:** It is very sensitive at identifying free sub-diaphragmatic gas (pneumoperitoneum) and has a much lower radiation dose than an abdominal radiograph. Erect chest X-ray should always be requested alongside a supine AXR in case of suspected perforation.

Abdominal X-rays for Medical Students, First Edition. Christopher G.D. Clarke and Anthony E.W. Dux.
© 2015 John Wiley & Sons, Ltd. Published 2015 by John Wiley & Sons, Ltd.

Radiograph quality

The quality of abdominal radiographs can vary widely. Before you think about the possible abnormalities on an abdominal radiograph, you must first assess the technical quality to ensure the image is adequate. The main questions to ask yourself are 'has everything been included on the radiograph?' and 'is the exposure adequate?'

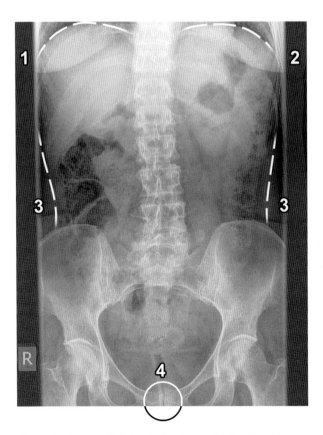

Figure 5: A normal abdominal radiograph showing the superior aspect of the liver (1), superior aspect of the spleen (2) and lateral abdominal walls (3) marked with dashed white lines. The pubic symphysis (4) is marked with a white circle (although ideally I would also like to see the inferior aspect of the pubic symphysis).

Inclusion

The entire anatomy should be included from the hemi-diaphragms to the symphysis pubis.
- The superior aspect of the liver (**1**) and spleen (**2**) should be included at the top of the radiograph.
- The lateral abdominal walls (**3**) should be seen on either side of the radiograph.
- The pubic symphysis (**4**) should be clearly visualised at the bottom of the radiograph.

Note: The average detector used to image the abdomen is slightly smaller than the average normal adult abdomen. Often two radiographs are needed to image the entire abdomen. In obese patients, sometimes the radiographs have to be used in the 'landscape' orientation rather than the traditional 'portrait' orientation to include everything.

Exposure

Exposure refers to the number of X-rays that reach the detector and make the image. An underexposed radiograph has not received enough X-rays and appears white/lighter. An overexposed radiograph has received too many X-rays and appears darker.

Abdominal X-rays for Medical Students, First Edition. Christopher G.D. Clarke and Anthony E.W. Dux.
© 2015 John Wiley & Sons, Ltd. Published 2015 by John Wiley & Sons, Ltd.

Exposure is less of a problem nowadays as inadequate images are usually terminated by the radiographer and repeated. Also, when viewing the radiograph, the contrast and brightness can be changed to compensate for poor exposure. However, under-exposure in obese patients can remain a problem and may limit the diagnostic value of the radiograph. To check the exposure is adequate, ensure the spine can be clearly visualised. Over-exposure is rarely an issue.

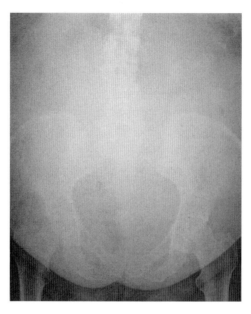

Figure 6: An underexposed abdominal radiograph demonstrating poor visualisation of the spine. It is more difficult to make out the bowel gas and the diagnostic value of this radiograph may be somewhat limited.

Normal anatomy on an abdominal X-ray

The following normal abdominal radiographs show the normal abdominal anatomy.

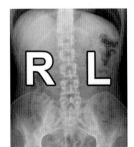

Right and left (Figure 7)

Remember, as you look at an abdominal radiograph the left side of the image is the patient's right side, and the right side of the image is the patient's left side. Always describe findings according to the patient's side.

Figure 7

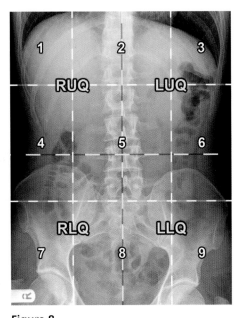

Quadrants and regions (Figure 8)

The abdomen can be divided into four quadrants or nine regions.
  The four quadrants (yellow dashed lines) are as follows:
  Right upper quadrant (RUQ); **left upper quadrant** (LUQ); **right lower quadrant** (RLQ); **left lower quadrant** (LLQ).
  The nine regions (white dashed lines) are as follows:

1. **Right hypochondriac**
2. **Epigastric**
3. **Left hypochondriac**
4. **Right lumbar**
5. **Umbilical**
6. **Left lumbar**
7. **Right iliac**
8. **Suprapubic**
9. **Left iliac**

Figure 8

Abdominal viscera 1 (Figure 9)

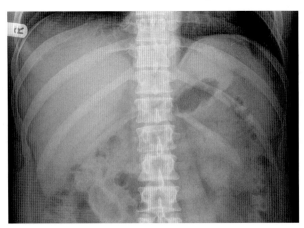
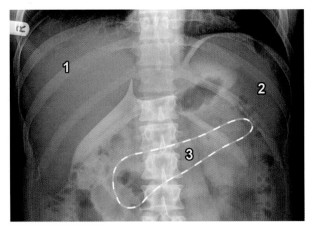

Figure 9

Abdominal X-rays for Medical Students, First Edition. Christopher G.D. Clarke and Anthony E.W. Dux.
© 2015 John Wiley & Sons, Ltd. Published 2015 by John Wiley & Sons, Ltd.

1. **Liver** (purple)
2. **Spleen** (pink)
3. **Location of the pancreas** (white outline) – not normally visualised

Abdominal viscera 2 (Figure 10)

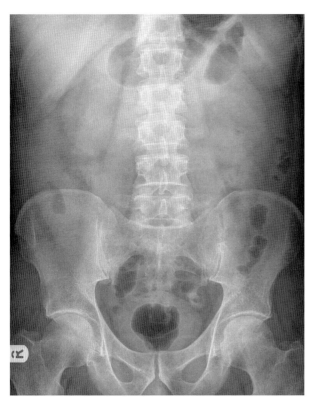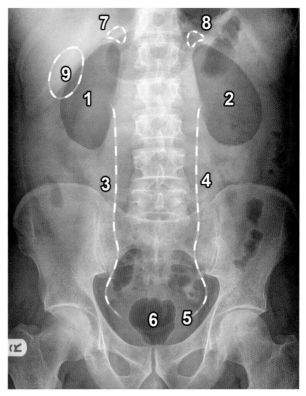

Figure 10

1. **Right kidney** (red)
2. **Left kidney** (red)
3. **Location of right ureter** (white outline) – not normally visualised
4. **Location of left ureter** (white outline) – not normally visualised
5. **Urinary bladder** (orange)

6. **Gas in the rectum** (green)
7. **Location of right adrenal gland** (white outline) – not normally visualised
8. **Location of left adrenal gland** (white outline) – not normally visualised
9. **Location of the gallbladder** (white outline) – not normally visualised

Note: The position of the gallbladder can be very variable. It can appear anywhere in the region of the right upper quadrant. The most common position (at the lower border of the liver) is shown in the earlier example.

Skeletal structures (Figure 11)

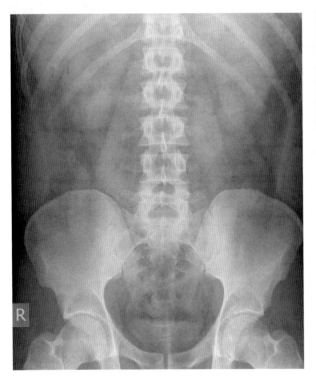
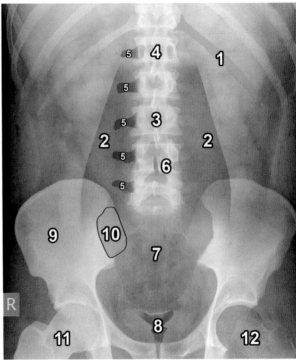

Figure 11

1. **Left 12th rib** (light green)
2. **Psoas outline** – left and right (red)
3. **Vertebral body of L3** (light blue)
4. **Pedicles of L1 vertebra** (orange)
5. **Right transverse processes of L1–L5** (black)
6. **Spinous process of L4** (brown)
7. **Sacrum** (blue)

8. **Coccyx** (rose)
9. **Right hemi-pelvis** (yellow)
10. **Right sacroiliac joint** (green)
11. **Right femur** (pink)
12. **Left femur** (purple)

Pelvis (Figure 12)

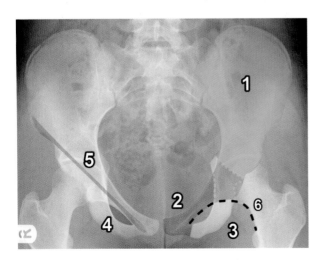

Figure 12

1. **Ilium** (green)
2. **Pubis** (red)
3. **Ischium** (yellow)
4. **Obturator foramen** (purple)
5. **Location of right inguinal ligament** (blue) – not normally visualised. The inguinal ligament runs between the anterior superior iliac spine and pubic tubercle
6. **Shenton's line** (black outline) – imaginary line along the inferior border of the superior pubic ramus and inferomedial border of the neck of femur

Lung bases (may be visualised at the top of the abdomen) (Figure 13)

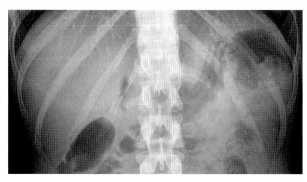
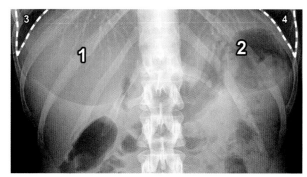

Figure 13

1. **Right lung base** (blue) – seen projected behind the liver
2. **Left lung base** (blue) – seen projected behind the stomach/spleen
3. **Right costophrenic angle** (white outline)
4. **Left costophrenic angle** (white outline)

Note: If you look carefully at the lung bases, you can often see the pulmonary vasculature as branching linear opacities (as seen in the earlier example).

Bowel 1 (Figure 14)

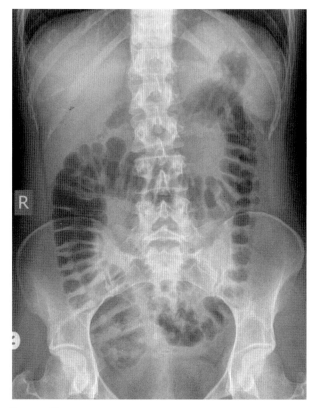
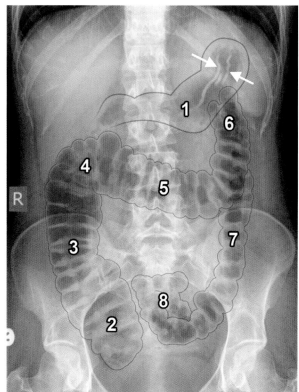

Figure 14

1. **Stomach** – note the stomach wall rugae (highlighted between the white arrows)
2. **Caecum**
3. **Ascending colon**
4. **Hepatic flexure**
5. **Transverse colon**
6. **Splenic flexure**
7. **Descending colon**
8. **Sigmoid colon**

Bowel 2 (Figure 15)

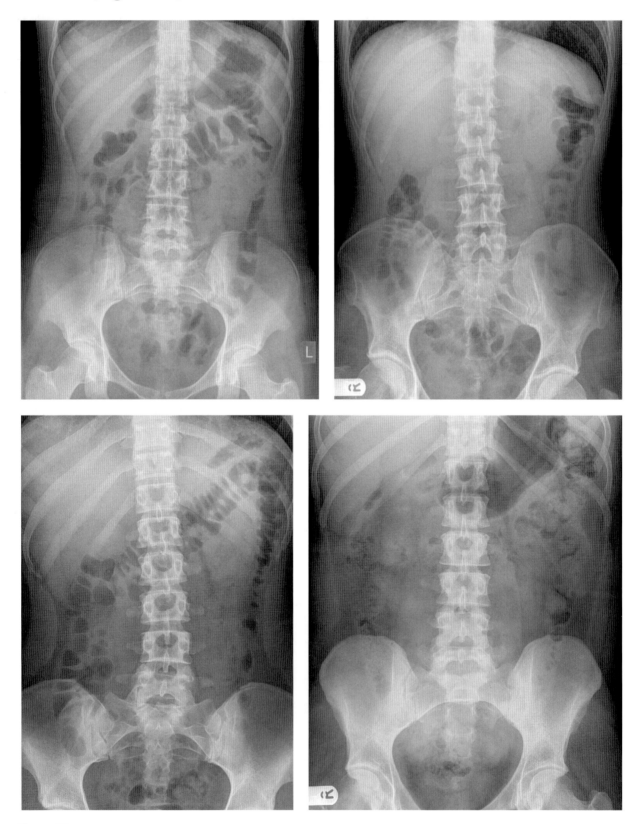

Figure 15

Four different normal abdominal radiographs showing examples of the normal variation in bowel gas pattern. Normally most of the bowel contains fluid/faeces (light grey) and therefore is not visualised on the radiograph. It is only the segments of bowel containing pockets of gas (black) that are visualised. The colon is more likely to contain gas than the small bowel and is therefore easier to visualise, as shown in the earlier examples.

The stomach is visible if it contains air; however, it may not be visible if it contains fluid or is empty. The small bowel air content is very variable depending on when the patient last ate, and can be pronounced when the patient is in pain due to air swallowing.

Presenting an abdominal radiograph

Be systematic!

You should present an abdominal radiograph in a systematic way to ensure you cover all areas and do not miss anything important. This is how you should present:

1. Give the **type** of radiograph.
2. Give the patient's name.
3. Give the date the radiograph was taken.
4. Briefly assess the radiograph quality (*see pages 6–7*) to ensure it is adequate.
5. Run through the ABCDE of abdominal radiographs (*see page 15*).
6. Give a short summary at the end.

e.g. "This is an **AP supine abdominal radiograph** of John Smith, taken on the 1st of January, 2015."

Always remember to describe what you are seeing. A good way to think about this is to **imagine you are describing the X-ray to a colleague over the phone**. If you see something, you must say **where it is anatomically** and **what it looks like**.

There are 16 examples of describing an abdominal radiograph on pages 94–106.

Abdominal X-rays for Medical Students, First Edition. Christopher G.D. Clarke and Anthony E.W. Dux.
© 2015 John Wiley & Sons, Ltd. Published 2015 by John Wiley & Sons, Ltd.

Overview of the ABCDE of abdominal radiographs

It is important to use a systematic approach when looking at an abdominal radiograph. The following ABCDE approach is easy to remember, so when it comes to your exams and you have a moment of panic after being asked to talk about an abdominal X-ray, you can stick to these basics, even if you don't have a clue what's going on!

A is for Air in the wrong place
- Look for pneumoperitoneum and pneumoretroperitoneum
- Look for gas in the biliary tree and portal vein

B is for Bowel
- Look for dilated small and large bowel
- Look for a volvulus
- Look for a distended stomach
- Look for a hernia
- Look for evidence of bowel wall thickening

C is for Calcification
- Look for clinically significant calcified structures such as calcified gallstones, renal calculus, nephrocalcinosis, pancreatic calcification and an abdominal aortic aneurysm (AAA)
- Look for a foetus (females)
- Look for clinically insignificant calcified structures such as costal cartilage calcification, phleboliths, mesenteric lymph nodes, calcified fibroids, prostate calcification and vascular calcification

D is for Disability (bones and solid organs)
- Look at the bony skeleton for fractures and sclerotic/lytic bone lesions
- Look at the spine for vertebral body height, alignment, pedicles and a 'bamboo spine'
- Look for solid organ enlargement

E is for Everything else
- Look for evidence of previous surgery and other medical devices
- Look for foreign bodies
- Look at the lung bases

Abdominal X-rays for Medical Students, First Edition. Christopher G.D. Clarke and Anthony E.W. Dux.
© 2015 John Wiley & Sons, Ltd. Published 2015 by John Wiley & Sons, Ltd.

A – Air in the wrong place

How to look?

- Look for free gas in the **peritoneal cavity** (pneumoperitoneum). To do this, look for **Rigler's sign** (gas present on both sides of the intestinal wall), **gas outlining the liver** and look to see if the **falciform ligament** is visible.
- Look for free gas in the **retroperitoneum** (pneumoretroperitoneum). To do this, look specifically for gas outlining the **kidneys**.
- Look at the **liver** (right upper quadrant) for linear areas of increased lucency. Gas seen towards the **centre of the liver** indicates gas in the **biliary tree (pneumobilia)**, for example within the common bile duct (CBD), hepatic ducts and/or gallbladder. Gas seen towards the **periphery of the liver** indicates gas in the **portal vein**.

What to look for in A – Air in the wrong place?

Abdominal X-rays for Medical Students, First Edition. Christopher G.D. Clarke and Anthony E.W. Dux.
© 2015 John Wiley & Sons, Ltd. Published 2015 by John Wiley & Sons, Ltd.

B – Bowel

How to look?
- Look at the bowel loops for **small** or **large bowel dilatation**.
- Look for a very large dilated loop of bowel that could represent a **sigmoid** or **caecal volvulus**. If the dilated bowel loop is in the upper abdomen, consider whether it may represent a **distended stomach**.
- Look at the left and right iliac regions for any bowel gas seen projected below the level of the inguinal ligament suggesting an **inguinal** or **femoral hernia**.
- Look for **thickening** of the **bowel wall** to suggest bowel wall inflammation. Specifically look for **thumbprinting** and the characteristic **lead pipe** colon.

What to look for in B – Bowel?

Abdominal X-rays for Medical Students, First Edition. Christopher G.D. Clarke and Anthony E.W. Dux.
© 2015 John Wiley & Sons, Ltd. Published 2015 by John Wiley & Sons, Ltd.

C – Calcification

How to look?

1. Look at the right upper quadrant for **calcified gallstones** (blue).
2. Look over the course of the kidneys and ureters for **renal stones** (green) and look specifically in the region of both kidneys for a **staghorn calculus** or **nephrocalcinosis** (light green).
3. Look at the suprapubic region for **bladder stones** (yellow).
4. Look at the upper central abdomen for **pancreatic calcification** (light blue).
5. Look in the regions of the upper poles of both kidneys for **adrenal calcification** (pink).
6. Look at the umbilical region for **abdominal aortic aneurysm (AAA) calcification** (red).

- In a female patient, look for a **foetus** ('skeleton with the abdomen' appearance).

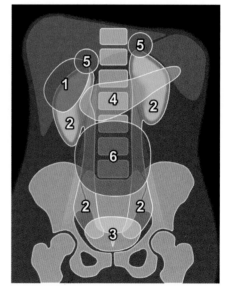

Figure 16: Diagrammatic representation of key areas to review when looking for abnormal calcification.

What to look for in C – Calcification?

Abdominal X-rays for Medical Students, First Edition. Christopher G.D. Clarke and Anthony E.W. Dux.
© 2015 John Wiley & Sons, Ltd. Published 2015 by John Wiley & Sons, Ltd.

D – Disability (bones and solid organs)

How to look?

- Look at the bony pelvis for a **fracture** (#). If a fracture is seen, use the **3 Polo rings test** to look for a second fracture (or disruption of the pubic symphysis or sacroiliac joints).
- Look for a **sclerotic** (increased density) or **lucent** (reduced density) bone lesion.
- Look at the spine for loss of **vertebral body height**, loss of visualisation of a **pedicle**, loss of normal **alignment** (e.g. scoliosis) and **bamboo spine** (ankylosing spondylitis).
- Look over the whole radiograph for any evidence of **solid organ enlargement**.

What to look for in D – Disability (bones and soft tissues)?

Abdominal X-rays for Medical Students, First Edition. Christopher G.D. Clarke and Anthony E.W. Dux.
© 2015 John Wiley & Sons, Ltd. Published 2015 by John Wiley & Sons, Ltd.

E – Everything else

How to look?
- Look at the whole radiograph for any evidence of previous surgery such as **surgical staples**, **clips**, **hernia clips** or **bowel anastomoses**.
- Look for any **catheters**, **drains**, **stents** or other **tubing** (e.g. gastric band or gastrostomy feeding tube).
- Look in the pelvis for an **intra-uterine device (IUD)** or **pessary**.
- Look carefully for any **foreign bodies**.
- Look at the **lung bases** for lung metastasis or other lung pathology.

What to look for in E – Everything else?

Abdominal X-rays for Medical Students, First Edition. Christopher G.D. Clarke and Anthony E.W. Dux.
© 2015 John Wiley & Sons, Ltd. Published 2015 by John Wiley & Sons, Ltd.

Pneumoperitoneum (gas in the peritoneal cavity)

Pneumoperitoneum literally means **free gas in the peritoneal cavity**. It usually indicates **bowel perforation**. Free gas may also be seen up to 3 weeks after abdominal surgery and in trauma (e.g. stabbing).

Main causes of pneumoperitoneum:
1. Perforated peptic ulcer
2. Perforated appendix/bowel diverticulum
3. Post-surgery
4. Trauma

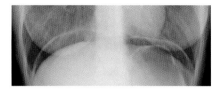

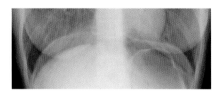

Figure 17: Two identical erect radiographs of the lower chest. The lower radiograph shows the pneumoperitoneum marked in turquoise.

Note: An abdominal radiograph and an erect chest radiograph are requested together when looking for a pneumoperitoneum. This is because an erect chest radiograph is very sensitive for detecting free abdominal gas since it can detect as little as 2–3 ml. On an erect chest X-ray the free gas is seen as a rim of blackness beneath and very closely opposed to the curve of the diaphragm.

The radiological signs of a pneumoperitoneum are as follows:
- **Rigler's sign:** Also known as the **double-wall sign**, this is seen when gas is present on both sides of the intestinal wall (i.e. gas within the bowel *and* free gas in the peritoneal cavity).

   Normally the bowel wall is only just visible, outlined by the gas within the bowel and peritoneal fat outside of the bowel. With a pneumoperitoneum the bowel wall is easily seen as it is outlined by gas within the bowel and gas outside of the bowel.

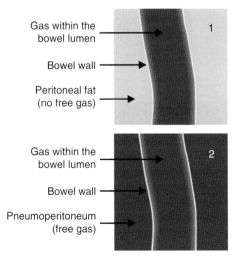

Figure 18: 1. Diagrammatic representation of normal appearances of the bowel wall. The lumen of the bowel contains gas. You can see the bowel wall, but there is little contrast between the bowel wall and the peritoneal fat outside of the bowel. **2.** Diagrammatic representation of **Rigler's sign** (double-wall sign). The lumen of the bowel contains gas, and there is also gas within the peritoneal cavity. The bowel wall is therefore clearly seen outlined by the gas either side.

Note: Rigler's sign is completely different to Rigler's triad. Please try not to confuse them. Rigler's triad refers to the three findings seen in a gallstone ileus (see page 33).

A

Note: Sometimes two loops of bowel lying next to each other can appear similar to Rigler's sign. Please be aware of this and look for loops of bowel, which can usually be identified by the presence of haustra (see page 34) or valvulae conniventes (see page 30).

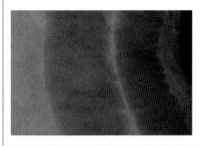 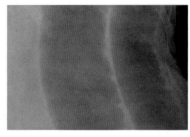

Figure 19: Two identical radiographs showing two loops of bowel adjacent to each other. This is not Rigler's sign because you can see the haustra within both loops of bowel. The right radiograph shows the bowel loops marked in brown.

- **Gas outlining the liver:** The liver edge may become easily visible due to surrounding free intra-peritoneal gas. Normally the liver (light grey) is outlined by peritoneal fat (dark grey). However, if there is a pneumoperitoneum, the liver is outlined by gas (black) giving a much greater contrast and therefore better visualisation of the liver edge.

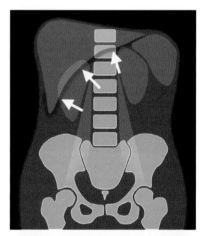

Figure 20: Diagrammatic representation of gas outlining the liver. When free gas is present in the peritoneal cavity, the liver edge is seen much more easily. The position of the liver edge is shown by the white arrows.

- **Falciform ligament sign:** The falciform ligament is a ligament attaching the liver to the anterior abdominal wall (a remnant of the umbilical vein). Normally it is not visible; however, the ligament may become visible if outlined by free intra-peritoneal gas either side of it in a supine patient.

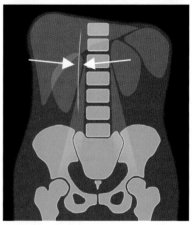

Figure 21: Diagrammatic representation of the falciform ligament sign. When free gas is present in the peritoneal cavity and the patient is lying supine, the falciform ligament becomes visible in the right upper quadrant as an opaque line extending inferiorly from the liver. This line appears in the position as shown by the white arrows.

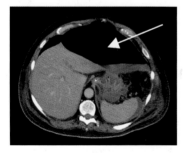

Note: If an abdominal radiograph and erect chest radiograph have been performed and there is still uncertainty about the diagnosis of pneumoperitoneum, a computed tomography (CT) scan of the abdomen should be requested. A CT scan gives a much higher radiation dose to the patient, but will clearly show the presence of free gas (white arrow) and may diagnose the underlying cause. Nowadays, most unwell patients with suspected pneumoperitoneum will go straight for a CT scan.

Figure 22: A CT slice through the abdomen showing a pneumoperitoneum. The gas is marked with an arrow.

Example 1

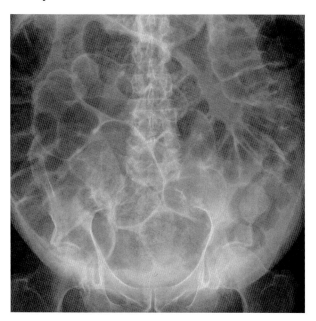
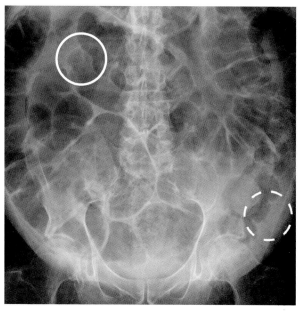

Figure 23: Two identical abdominal radiographs showing a pneumoperitoneum. There are loops of bowel with gas outlining both sides of the bowel wall in keeping with Rigler's sign. The right radiograph shows in turquoise and brown the areas where Rigler's sign is most clearly seen. The lumen of the bowel is marked in brown and the free gas outlining the bowel wall marked in turquoise. The best example of Rigler's sign is marked with a white circle. An area of normal appearing bowel wall is marked with a white dashed circle for comparison. (You can also see dilated loops of large bowel.)

Example 2

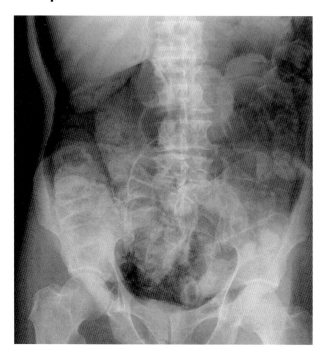
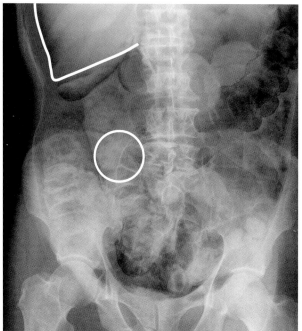

Figure 24: Two identical abdominal radiographs showing a large pneumoperitoneum. There are loops of bowel with gas outlining both sides of the bowel wall in keeping with Rigler's sign. The right radiograph shows in turquoise the areas where the pneumoperitoneum is most clearly seen. Where Rigler's sign is most clearly seen, the lumen of the bowel is marked in brown. The best example of Rigler's sign is marked with a white circle. You can also see gas outlining the liver as shown by the white line.

Example 3

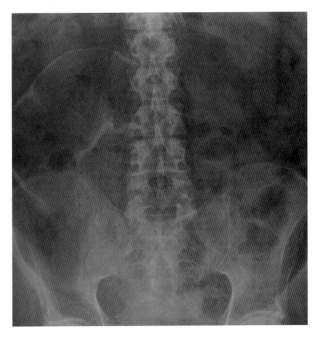
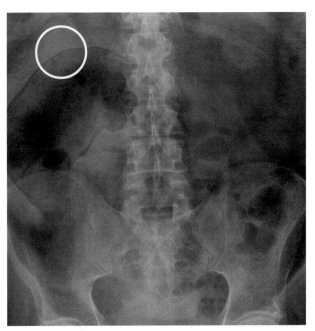

Figure 25: Two identical abdominal radiographs showing a pneumoperitoneum. There is a dilated loop of bowel with gas outlining both sides of the bowel wall in keeping with Rigler's sign. The right radiograph shows in turquoise and brown the areas where Rigler's sign is most clearly seen. The lumen of the bowel is marked in brown and the free gas outlining the bowel wall marked in turquoise. The best example of Rigler's sign is marked with a white circle.

Example 4

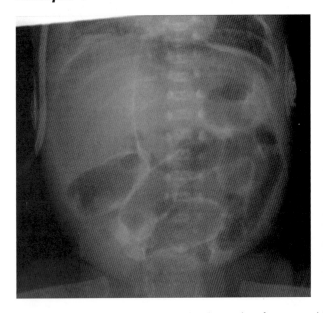
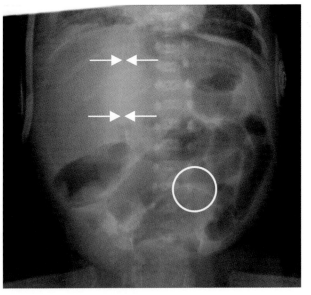

Figure 26: Two identical abdominal radiographs of a young child showing a pneumoperitoneum. There are loops of bowel with gas outlining both sides of the bowel wall in keeping with Rigler's sign, and there is gas outlining the falciform ligament in keeping with the falciform ligament sign. The right radiograph shows in turquoise and brown the areas where Rigler's sign is most clearly seen. The lumen of the bowel is marked in brown and the free gas outlining the bowel wall marked in turquoise. The position of the falciform ligament is shown with white arrows. The best example of Rigler's sign is marked with a white circle. (You can also see dilated loops of bowel.)

Example 5

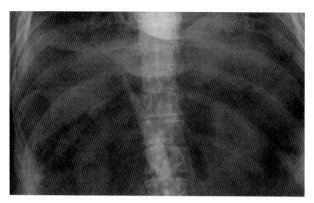
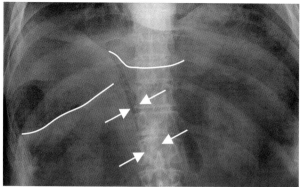

Figure 27: Two identical abdominal radiographs of the upper abdomen showing a pneumoperitoneum. There is gas outlining the falciform ligament in keeping with the falciform ligament sign and there is also gas outlining the liver. The right radiograph shows in turquoise the areas where the pneumoperitoneum is most clearly seen. The position of the falciform ligament is shown with white arrows and the outline of the liver edge is shown by the white lines.

Example 6

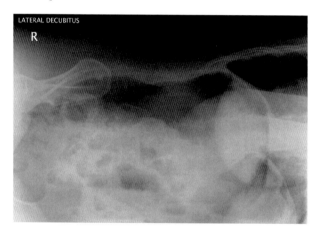
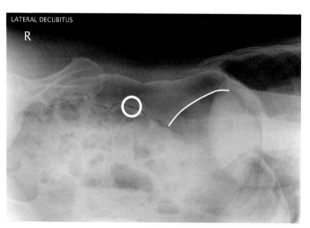

Figure 28: Two identical abdominal radiographs taken in the left lateral decubitus position showing a large pneumoperitoneum. The patient is lying on their left side. You can see the bony pelvis on the left of the image, and the dark area on the top right of the image is the base of the patient's right lung. There are loops of bowel with gas outlining both sides of the bowel wall in keeping with Rigler's sign and there is also gas outlining the liver. The right radiograph shows in turquoise the areas where the pneumoperitoneum is most clearly seen. Where Rigler's sign is most clearly seen, the lumen of the bowel is marked in brown. The best example of Rigler's sign is marked with a white circle. You can also see gas outlining the liver as shown by the white line. The right lung is marked in blue.

Pneumoretroperitoneum (gas in the retroperitoneal space)

Pneumoretroperitoneum literally means **gas in the retroperitoneal space**. It is rarely seen but is always abnormal.

The retroperitoneal space is a potential space within the abdominal cavity retro (behind) to the peritoneum. It contains the kidneys, ureters, adrenal glands, aorta, inferior vena cava (IVC), most of the pancreas and duodenum, and the ascending and descending colon.

Main causes of retroperitoneal gas:

1. **Bowel perforation**
   - Posterior duodenal perforation (e.g. peptic ulcer perforation/post-ERCP [endoscopic retrograde cholangio pancreatography] or post-sphincterotomy)
   - Ascending or descending colon perforation (e.g. carcinoma/diverticulitis/ischaemic colitis)
   - Rectal perforation (e.g. post-surgery/post-endoscopy/foreign body insertion)
2. **Post-surgical** (e.g. residual air from urological/adrenal/spinal surgery)

On an abdominal radiograph the gas outlines retroperitoneal structures such as the kidneys, psoas muscles and retroperitoneal bowel (duodenum, ascending colon, descending colon and rectum). At first glance a pneumoretroperitoneum can appear similar to a pneumoperitoneum as both give increased gas (blackness) on an abdominal radiograph.

The key to identifying a pneumoretroperitoneum is to look for **gas (blackness) surrounding all or part of the kidneys**.

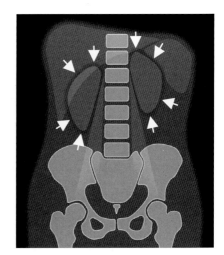

Figure 29: Diagrammatic representation of the appearance of retroperitoneal gas outlining the kidneys. When gas is present in the retroperitoneal space the kidney edges are seen much more easily. The position of the kidney edges are shown by the white arrows.

Note: It is possible to have both a pneumoretroperitoneum and pneumoperitoneum at the same time. Remember the key to identifying retroperitoneal gas is to look for gas surrounding the kidneys. In pneumoperitoneum alone you will not see the kidneys.

Example 1

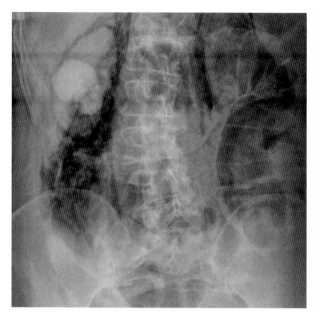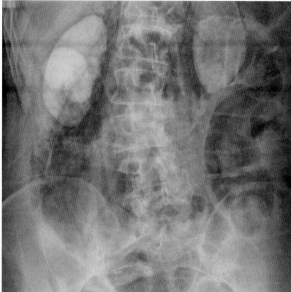

Figure 30: Two identical abdominal radiographs showing gas in the retroperitoneal space. There are patchy areas of blackness (gas) seen outlining both kidneys either side of the spine. The right radiograph shows the retroperitoneal gas marked in turquoise, clearly outlining both kidneys.

Example 2

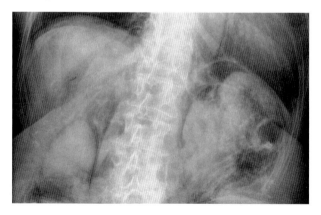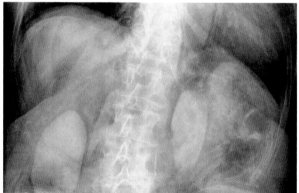

Figure 31: Two identical abdominal radiographs of the upper abdomen showing gas in the retroperitoneal space. There are patchy areas of blackness (gas) seen outlining both kidneys either side of the spine. The right radiograph shows the retroperitoneal gas marked in turquoise, clearly outlining both kidneys.

Pneumobilia (gas in the biliary tree)

Pneumobilia is **gas** in the **biliary tree**. It appears as **branching dark lines** in the **centre** of the **liver**, usually larger and more prominent towards the hilum. Sometimes you can also see gas in the common bile duct.

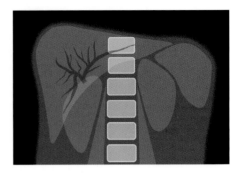

Figure 32: Diagrammatic representation of the appearance of gas in the biliary tree on a plain abdominal radiograph. The gas appears as a linear branching pattern (like a tree) and is seen in the centre of the liver, becoming more prominent towards the hilum.

Note: Pneumobilia can appear very similar to portal venous gas as both give a branching gas pattern within the liver. The way to tell them apart is to look at the location of the gas. Gas in the biliary tree (pneumobilia) is seen in the centre (hilum) of the liver, not the periphery. Portal venous gas is seen in the periphery of the liver because blood in the portal vein flows from the centre (hilum) towards the periphery.

There are many causes of pneumobilia, not all of which are pathological. The main causes are as follows:
1. **Recent ERCP/incompetent sphincter of Oddi** (e.g. post-sphincterotomy)
2. **External biliary drain insertion/biliary stent insertion**
3. **Biliary-enteric connection** (abnormal connection between biliary tree and bowel)
   - Surgical anastomosis (e.g. Whipple's procedure)
   - Spontaneous (e.g. gallstone ileus)
4. **Infection (rare)**
   - Emphysematous cholecystitis (acute cholecystitis with gas-forming organism)

Example

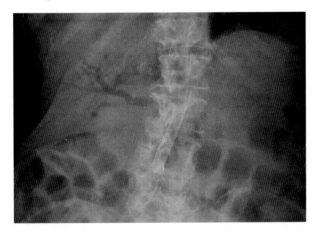
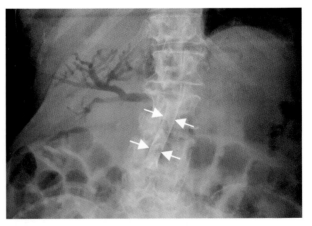

Figure 33: Two identical abdominal radiographs of the upper abdomen showing gas within the biliary tree. There are branching dark lines (gas) projected over the centre of the liver, larger and more prominent towards the hilum. There is also a biliary stent projected over the midline (arrows). This is situated within the common bile duct and explains why gas is easily able to travel from the duodenum into the biliary system. The presence of pneumobilia indicates that the stent is probably patent. The right radiograph shows the gas within the biliary tree marked in dark blue.

A

Portal venous gas (gas in the portal vein)

Gas in the portal vein appears as **branching dark lines** within the **periphery** of the **liver** on a plain abdominal radiograph. In adults, it indicates serious intra-abdominal pathology and is associated with a very high mortality rate. In infants it is a finding of far less consequence.

Main causes of gas in the portal vein:

1. **Ischaemic bowel** (most common)
2. **Necrotising enterocolitis (NEC)** (most common in an infant)
3. **Severe intra-abdominal sepsis** (diverticulitis/pelvic abscess/appendicitis)

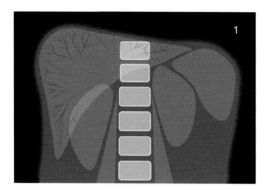
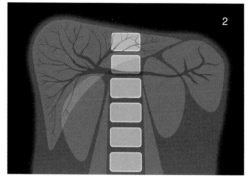

Figure 34: Diagrammatic representation of the appearance of portal venous gas on a plain abdominal radiograph. The gas appears as a linear branching pattern in the periphery of the liver (**1**). This is because the portal venous blood flows from the portal vein towards the periphery of the liver. If there is a large amount of gas in the portal vein, then it may be seen extending from the periphery to the centre of the liver and even within the splenic vein (**2**).

Note: Remember pneumobilia can appear very similar to portal venous gas as both give a branching gas pattern within the liver. The way to tell them apart is to look at the location of the gas. Gas in the biliary tree (pneumobilia) is seen in the centre (hilum) of the liver, not the periphery. Portal venous gas is seen in the periphery of the liver because blood in the portal vein flows from the centre (hilum) towards the periphery.

Example

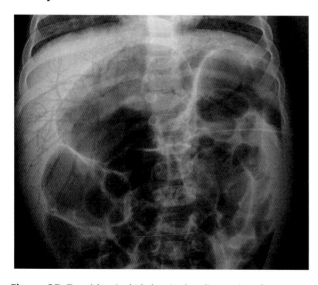
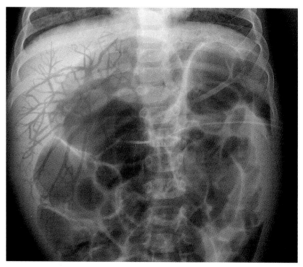

Figure 35: Two identical abdominal radiographs of a child showing gas in the portal venous system. There are branching dark lines (gas) projected over the periphery of the liver. In this case the gas is so extensive that it is also seen in splenic vein. The right radiograph shows the gas within the portal venous system marked in dark blue. Gas in the splenic vein is marked in light blue. (You can also see dilated loops of large bowel.)

Dilated small bowel

Distension of the small bowel is a sign of **mechanical obstruction** or **ileus**. In a normal individual the small bowel is not visualised because it is collapsed or contains fluid.

There are two main processes causing dilated small bowel:

1. **Mechanical obstruction:** Physical obstruction of the intestine preventing normal transit of digestive products. The bowel proximal to the obstruction is dilated. Therefore, the more distal the obstruction, the more loops of bowel are visible. Causes of mechanical obstruction are divided into acquired and congenital:

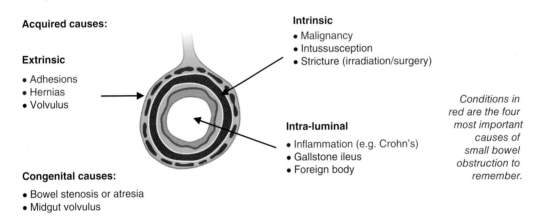

Acquired causes:

Extrinsic

- Adhesions
- Hernias
- Volvulus

Congenital causes:

- Bowel stenosis or atresia
- Midgut volvulus

Intrinsic

- Malignancy
- Intussusception
- Stricture (irradiation/surgery)

Intra-luminal

- Inflammation (e.g. Crohn's)
- Gallstone ileus
- Foreign body

Conditions in red are the four most important causes of small bowel obstruction to remember.

Figure 36: Causes of mechanical small bowel obstruction.

2. **Ileus:** Disruption of the normal propulsive ability of the gastrointestinal tract (i.e. failure of peristalsis). Causes include the following:
   - post-operative
   - intra-abdominal infection or inflammation
   - anti-cholinergic drugs

Mechanical obstruction and ileus appear **identical**, and in most cases the underlying cause cannot be determined on an abdominal X-ray. Radiological signs to look for include the following:

- **Dilation >3 cm:** The small bowel is dilated if it measures over 3 cm in diameter. *Note: The height of an adult vertebral body is approximately 4 cm. You can use this as a quick comparison to estimate the diameter of the bowel.*
- **Central location:** The dilated loops are more likely to be centrally located on the abdominal radiograph. *Note: Large bowel tends to be peripherally located.*
- **Valvulae conniventes:** These are the mucosal folds of the small intestine. They are thin, closely spaced and classically seen as a continuous thin line across the entire width of the bowel.

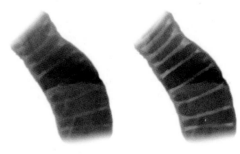

Figure 37: Two identical images showing a loop of dilated small bowel with the classical radiographic appearances of valvulae conniventes crossing the entire width of the bowel. The right image shows the valvulae conniventes highlighted in white.

Note: Sometimes dilated loops of bowel can contain fluid rather than gas, which can result in a normal-appearing abdominal radiograph.

Example 1

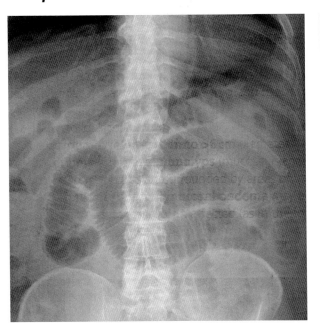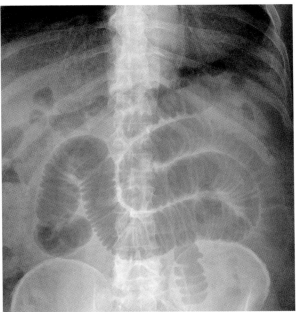

Figure 38: Two identical abdominal radiographs showing dilated small bowel. The bowel is visible as there is gas (black) within. You can tell that it is small bowel as it is centrally located and valvulae conniventes can be seen throughout. The loops measure >3 cm in diameter therefore they are dilated. The right radiograph shows the dilated small bowel marked in blue.

Example 2

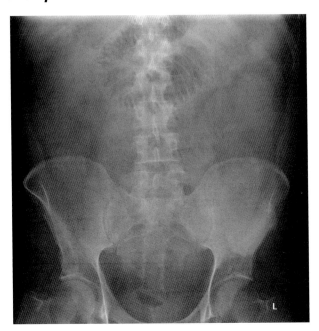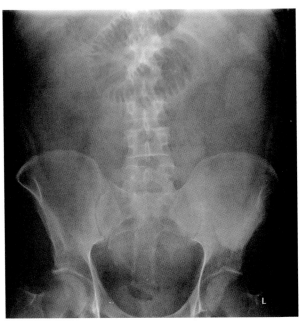

Figure 39: Two identical abdominal radiographs showing a loop of dilated small bowel. The loop of bowel is visible as there is gas (black) within. You can tell that it is small bowel as valvulae conniventes can be seen throughout. The loop measures >3 cm in diameter and is therefore dilated. When a single dilated loop is seen (as in this case) it is known as a **sentinel loop**. It is a feature that is occasionally due to a localised ileus from nearby inflammation causing local paralysis and accumulation of gas in the intestinal loop. The right radiograph shows the dilated small bowel marked in blue.

Example 3

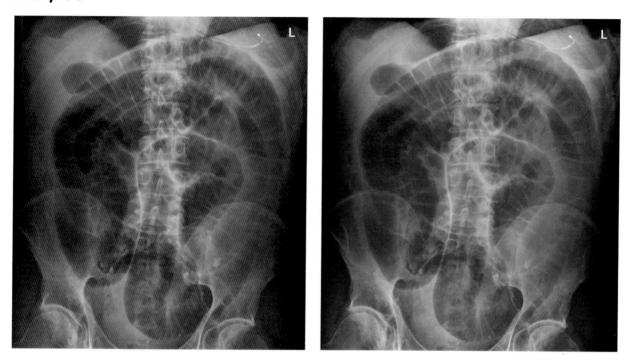

Figure 40: Two identical abdominal radiographs showing dilated small bowel. The small bowel is visible as there is gas (black) within. You can tell that it is small bowel as it is centrally located and valvulae conniventes can be seen throughout. The loops measure >3 cm in diameter and are therefore dilated. The right radiograph shows the dilated small bowel marked in blue. (You can also see a wire from an intra-cardiac device.)

Example 4

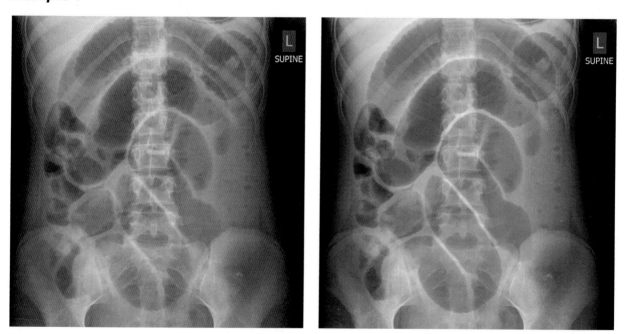

Figure 41: Two identical abdominal radiographs showing dilated small bowel. The small bowel is visible as there is gas (black) within. The loops of bowel are centrally located and valvulae conniventes are seen in the upper loops. The loops measure >3 cm in diameter and are therefore dilated. You can also see gas within the ascending colon, which is within normal limits. The right radiograph shows the dilated small bowel marked in blue.

Special Case: Gallstone ileus

A gallstone ileus is an uncommon cause of mechanical small bowel obstruction. Recurrent episodes of cholecystitis cause adhesion of the **gallbladder** to the **bowel** (usually duodenum) and eventually a **fistula** forms. A large gallstone then enters the bowel and causes **obstruction**, typically at the ileocecal valve.

A gallstone ileus gives the classical **Rigler's triad**:
1. **Pneumobilia**
2. **Small bowel obstruction**
3. **Gallstone** (usually in the right iliac fossa, but only seen in approximately 30% of cases)

> **Note:** Often the gallstone itself is not visualised as most gallstones are not calcified and therefore do not show up on an abdominal radiograph.

Example

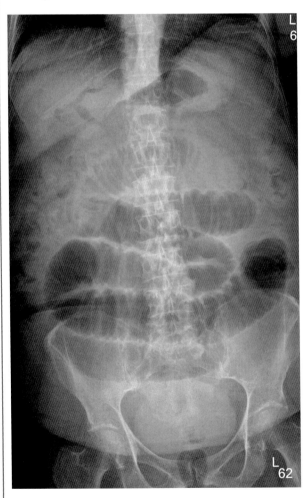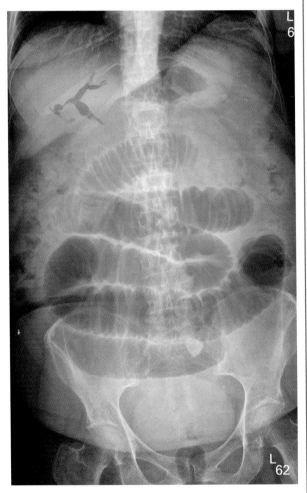

Figure 42: Two identical abdominal radiographs of a patient with a gallstone ileus. There are branching dark lines (gas) projected over the centre of the liver, larger and more prominent towards the hilum, in keeping with pneumobilia. There are centrally located loops of bowel measuring >3 cm in diameter with valvulae conniventes seen throughout, in keeping with dilated small bowel. There is a calcified opacity projected over the left sacrum in keeping with a large calcified gallstone. The right radiograph shows the pneumobilia marked in dark blue, dilated small bowel marked in blue and gallstone marked in yellow.

B

Dilated large bowel

Large bowel distension is almost always due to **large bowel obstruction**. The bowel proximal to the obstruction is dilated and the bowel distal to the obstruction is usually collapsed.

Causes of large bowel obstruction include the following:

- **Malignancy** (colorectal carcinoma is the most common cause of large bowel obstruction in adults)
- **Diverticular stricture**
- **Faecal impaction** (most common cause in immobile elderly persons)
- **Volvulus** (*please see pages 37–38 for examples*)

Radiographic appearances:

- **Dilation >5.5 cm:** The large bowel is dilated if it measures over 5.5 cm in diameter. The caecum is allowed to reach 9 cm before being called dilated.
- **Circumferential location:** The dilated loops are more likely to be peripherally located on the abdominal radiograph, surrounding the small bowel. The exception to this is that the transverse colon often loops down towards the pelvis and can cross the centre of the radiograph.
- **Haustra:** These are the small pouches in the wall of the large intestine. The taenia coli (ribbons of smooth muscle which run along the length of the colon) are shorter than the colon itself, therefore the colon becomes sacculated between the taenia coli forming the haustra. The lines between the haustra are called **haustral folds** and typically do not cross the entire width of the bowel (unlike valvulae conniventes).

> **Note:** If the bowel is grossly distended, then the haustra may not be seen.

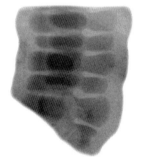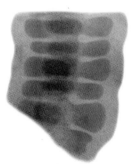

Figure 43: Two identical images showing a loop of dilated large bowel with the classical radiographic appearances of haustra. The right image shows the haustra highlighted in green.

Comparison of small and large bowel X-ray appearances

	Dilated small bowel	Dilated large bowel
Size	>3 cm (does not get larger than ~4 cm)	>5.5 cm >9 cm for the caecum
Position	Central	Circumferential/ peripheral location
Mucosal/wall pattern	Valvulae conniventes (*thin/closely spaced/cross the entire width of the bowel*)	Haustral folds (*thick/widely spaced/do not cross the entire width of the bowel*)

Example 1

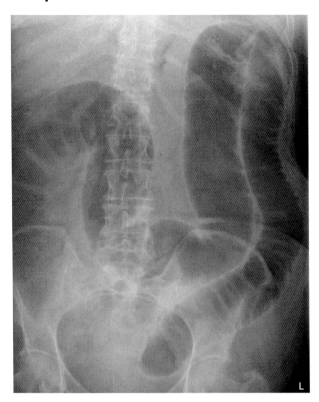
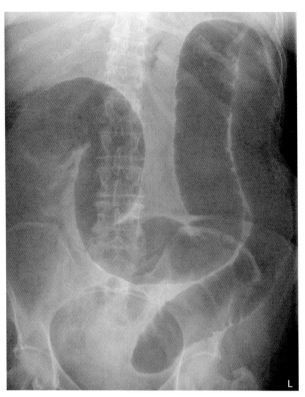

Figure 44: Two identical abdominal radiographs showing dilated large bowel. The large bowel is visible as there is gas (black) within. You can tell that it is large bowel as it is distended >5.5 cm, circumferentially located and haustra are seen within. The right radiograph shows the dilated large bowel marked in green.

Example 2

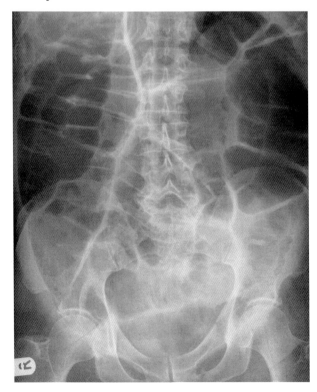
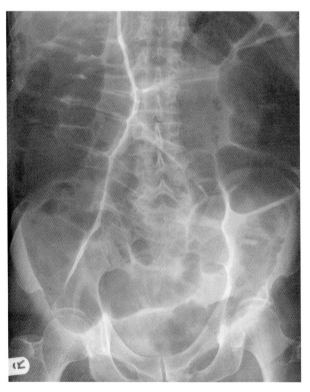

Figure 45: Two identical abdominal radiographs showing dilated large bowel. The large bowel is visible as there is gas (black) within. You can tell that it is large bowel as it is distended >5.5 cm (much larger than dilated small bowel would usually get) and haustra are seen within. The right radiograph shows the dilated large bowel marked in green.

Example 3

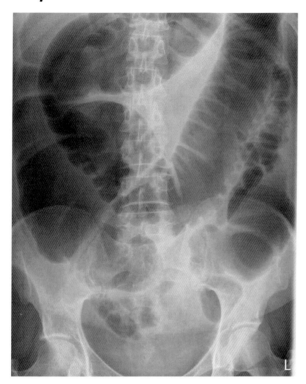
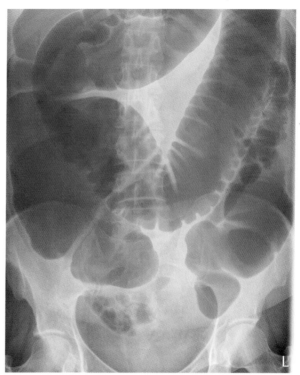

Figure 46: Two identical abdominal radiographs showing dilated large bowel. The large bowel is visible as there is gas (black) within. You can tell that it is large bowel as it is distended >5.5 cm, circumferentially located and haustra are seen within. The right radiograph shows the dilated large bowel marked in green.

Example 4

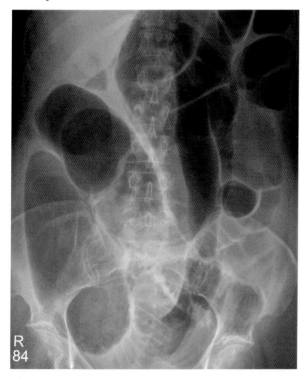
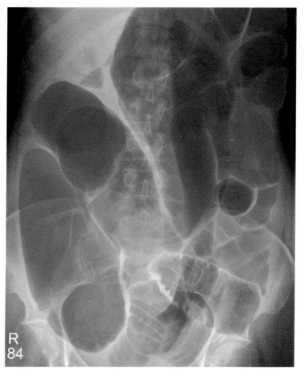

Figure 47: Two identical abdominal radiographs showing dilated large bowel and two loops of dilated small bowel. The bowel is visible as there is gas (black) within. The large bowel loops are distended >5.5 cm, circumferentially located and a few haustra are seen within. The two loops of distended small bowel are identified by the presence of valvulae conniventes and indicate incompetence of the ileocecal valve since gas has passed retrogradely from the large bowel into the small bowel. The right radiograph shows the dilated large bowel marked in green and the dilated small bowel marked in blue.

Volvulus

A volvulus is the **twisting of the bowel** on its **mesentery**. It causes partial or complete bowel obstruction. The two commonest types of volvulus in adults are **sigmoid volvulus** and **caecal volvulus**. A volvulus can give symptoms by two processes:
1. **Bowel obstruction:** The loop of twisted bowel causes a 'closed-loop' obstruction.
2. **Bowel ischaemia:** In some cases the twisting of the bowel mesentery compromises the vascular supply to the bowel leading to ischaemia and eventually necrosis, which can be fatal.

Sigmoid volvulus

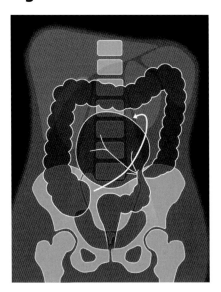

A sigmoid volvulus is caused when the **sigmoid colon twists** on its **mesentery**. It is usually seen in the elderly or institutionalised patients.

Radiological signs of a sigmoid volvulus:
1. **Coffee bean sign:** The shape of the distended gas filled 'closed loop' of colon looks like a large coffee bean.
2. **General lack of haustra:** Often the bowel is so distended that haustra flatten out and are no longer seen.
3. **Distension of the ascending, transverse and descending colon:** The colon proximal to the obstruction (volvulus) is often distended, but not always.

Figure 48: Diagrammatic representation of a sigmoid volvulus. The sigmoid colon has its own mesentery, which is liable to twisting causing obstruction and distension of the sigmoid colon with gas.

Caecal volvulus

A caecal volvulus is caused when the **caecal colon twists** on its **mesentery**. In most patients the caecum is a retroperitoneal structure, but in some patients the caecum is intraperitoneal with a mesentery. These patients have an increased risk of developing a caecal volvulus.

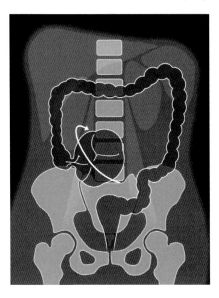

Radiological signs of a caecal volvulus:
1. **Comma shaped:** The shape of the distended gas filled 'closed loop' of colon often looks like a large comma (more rounded in shape than a sigmoid volvulus).
2. **Haustra often visible:** The haustral folds are often still clearly visualised, even when the bowel is very distended.
3. **Collapse of the ascending, transverse and descending colon:** The colon distal to the obstruction (volvulus) is often collapsed.

Figure 49: Diagrammatic representation of a caecal volvulus. The caecum has twisted causing obstruction and distension of the caecum with gas.

Sigmoid volvulus example 1

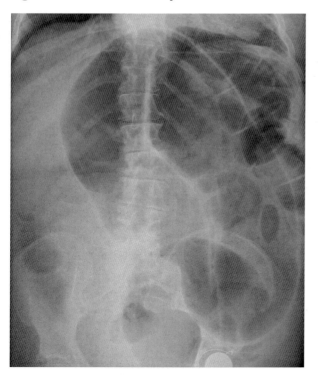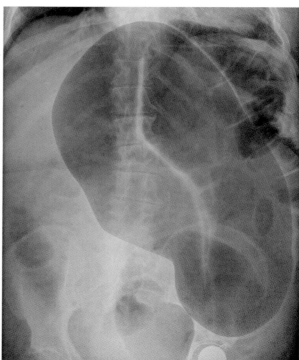

Figure 50: Two identical abdominal radiographs showing a sigmoid volvulus. There is a 'coffee bean'–shaped loop of distended bowel crossing the midline and extending to the right upper quadrant. There is a general lack of haustra. The proximal large bowel is somewhat distended secondary to the obstruction from the volvulus. The right radiograph shows the sigmoid volvulus marked in brown. (You can also see a left hip prosthesis.)

Sigmoid volvulus example 2

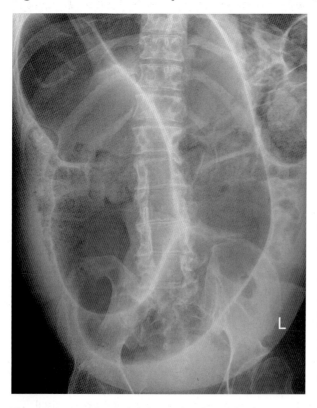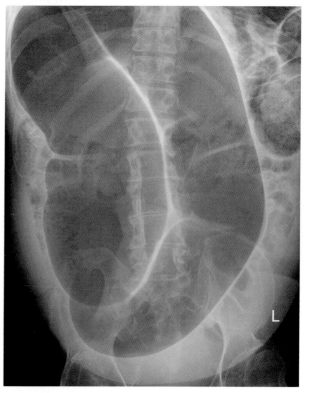

Figure 51: Two identical abdominal radiographs showing a sigmoid volvulus. There is a 'coffee bean'–shaped loop of distended bowel crossing the midline and extending to the right upper quadrant. There is a general lack of haustra. The right radiograph shows the sigmoid volvulus marked in brown.

Caecal volvulus example 1

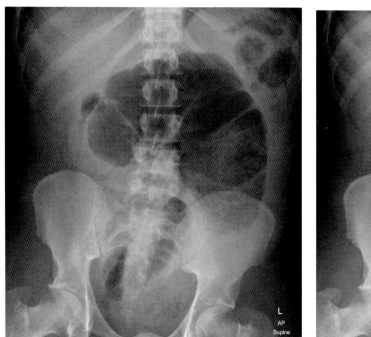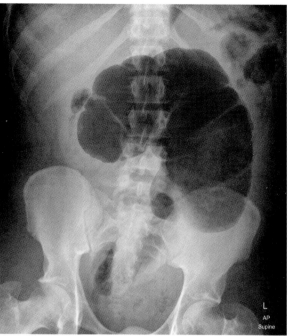

Figure 52: Two identical abdominal radiographs showing a caecal volvulus. There is a rounded comma-shaped loop of distended large bowel in the centre of the abdomen with haustra seen within. The remainder of the colon distal to the caecal volvulus (obstruction) is collapsed. The right radiograph shows the caecal volvulus marked in red.

Caecal volvulus example 2

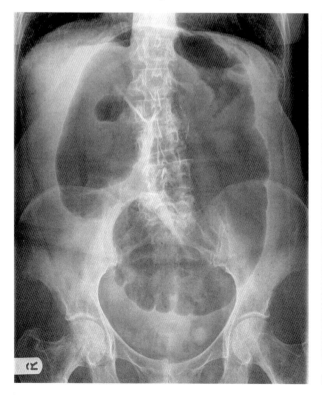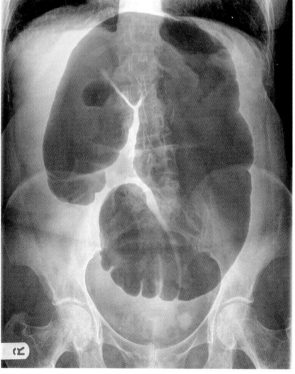

Figure 53: Two identical abdominal radiographs showing a caecal volvulus. There is a rounded comma-shaped loop of distended large bowel in the centre of the abdomen with a few haustra seen within. The remainder of the colon distal to the caecal volvulus (obstruction) is collapsed. The right radiograph shows the caecal volvulus marked in red.

Dilated stomach

The stomach may become overly distended if filled with gas or fluid.

Causes of gas filled stomach distension:
- **Bowel obstruction** (e.g. malignancy or scarring in the duodenum secondary to peptic ulcer disease)
- **Aerophagia (excessive air swallowing)** (e.g. distressed patients or as a side effect of non-invasive ventilation)

Causes of fluid-filled stomach distension:
- **Bowel obstruction** (e.g. malignancy or scarring in the duodenum secondary to peptic ulcer disease)
- **Chronic gastroparesis** (e.g. autonomic neuropathy from poorly controlled diabetes)

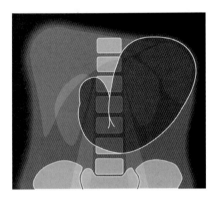

The radiological appearances are of a large stomach-shaped gas filled (dark) or fluid filled (light grey) loop in the upper abdomen. The stomach may be so distended that the normal rugae (*see page 11*) are not clearly seen.

Figure 54: Diagrammatic representation of the appearance of a dilated stomach full of gas. There is a large U-shaped or stomach-shaped loop of bowel in the left upper quadrant. If very large, the stomach can extend inferiorly over the centre of the abdomen.

Example

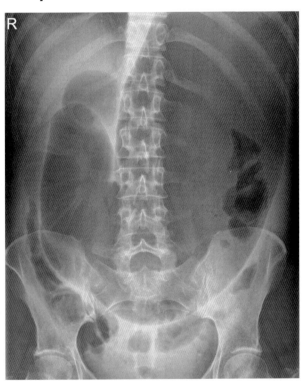
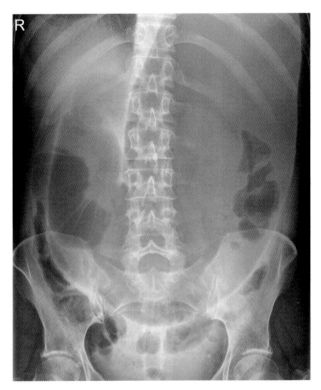

Figure 55: Two identical abdominal radiographs showing a gas-filled dilated stomach. There is a loop of stomach-shaped distended bowel in the upper abdomen. On the right side of the abdomen, you can see that the duodenum is partially distended as valvulae conniventes are seen. The findings are suggestive of a proximal small bowel obstruction, possibly in the region of the distal duodenum or proximal jejunum. The right radiograph shows the dilated stomach in light blue and the loop of duodenum in blue.

Hernia

A hernia is the **protrusion** of an **organ (or part of an organ)** through the **wall of the cavity containing it**.
On an abdominal radiograph the only hernias that can be easily identified are those of a **groin hernia (inguinal or femoral)** containing a loop of bowel which contains gas. If the loop of bowel contains fluid, it will not be easily seen.

If the lower pelvis is not included on an abdominal radiograph, then you will not be able to look for a groin hernia; however, if it is included, then a hernia is important to identify as it may be the cause of bowel obstruction.

Note: Hernias are usually an incidental finding on an abdominal radiograph.

B

Radiological appearances:
- **Loops of gas-filled bowel seen BELOW the level of the inguinal ligament**
  - A quick way to assess is to see if there are any loops of bowel projected over or below the obturator foramen.
- **Soft tissue swelling on the side of the hernia**
  - As well as loops of bowel (black), there is often also increased soft tissue swelling (light grey). This is due to the herniated mesenteric fat and/or oedema associated with the herniated loop of bowel.

Note: Hernias can occur in other locations such as around the umbilicus and at the site of previous surgery (incisional hernia), but these are very difficult to diagnose on an abdominal radiograph and most are not visualised at all.

Example 1

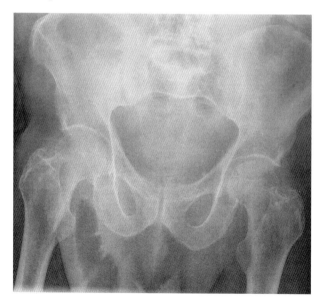 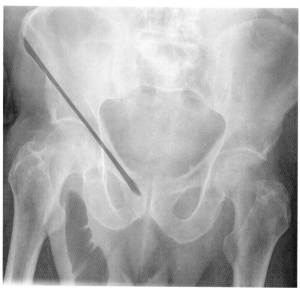

Figure 56: Two identical abdominal radiographs showing a right groin hernia. There is a loop of gas-filled bowel projected over the right groin area below the right obturator foramen and below the level of the inguinal ligament. The right radiograph shows the herniated loop of bowel in green and the position of the right inguinal ligament in grey.

Example 2

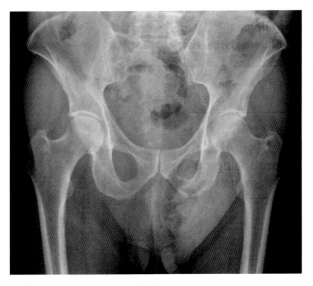 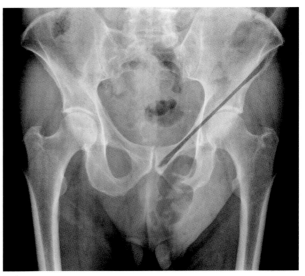

Figure 57: Two identical abdominal radiographs showing a left groin hernia. There is a loop of gas-filled bowel projected over the left groin area over and below the left obturator foramen and below the level of the inguinal ligament. The right radiograph shows the herniated loop of bowel in green and the position of the left inguinal ligament in grey.

Example 3

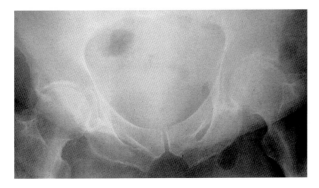 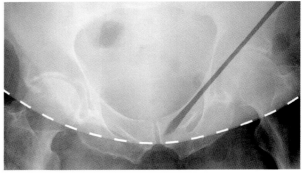

Figure 58: Two identical abdominal radiographs showing a left groin hernia. There is a loop of gas-filled bowel projected over the left groin area below the left obturator foramen and below the level of the inguinal ligament. The right radiograph shows the herniated loop of bowel in green and the position of the left inguinal ligament in grey. The white dotted line indicates the position of overhanging anterior abdominal wall in this overweight patient.

Bowel wall inflammation

Bowel wall inflammation can occur anywhere along the bowel, but is most commonly seen in the **large bowel**. Inflammation of the large bowel is termed **colitis**.

Main causes of colitis:
- **Inflammatory bowel disease** (e.g. ulcerative colitis or Crohn's disease)
- **Ischaemic bowel**
- **Infection** (e.g. pseudomembranous colitis from *Clostridium difficile*)

> **Note:** It is impossible to differentiate between the different causes of colitis using a plain abdominal radiograph; however, remember that ulcerative colitis only affects the large bowel, Crohn's and infection may affect anywhere along the gastrointestinal tract and ischaemic bowel usually affects a specific vascular territory (e.g. superior mesenteric artery territory [midgut] or inferior mesenteric artery territory [hindgut]).

Radiological signs of bowel wall inflammation:
1. **Bowel wall thickening:** Inflammation causes mucosal oedema and therefore thickening of the bowel wall. Often you can see the thickened bowel wall outlined by gas within the bowel lumen and peritoneal fat outside of the bowel.
   - **'Thumbprinting':** Mucosal oedema may cause severe thickening of the haustral folds of the colon, such that the folds appear as 'thumb-shaped' projections into the bowel lumen.

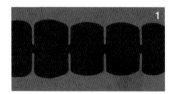

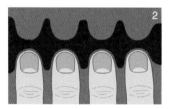

Figure 59: 1. Diagrammatic representation of normal appearances of the colonic bowel wall with thin haustral folds projecting into the bowel lumen. **2.** Diagrammatic representation of the appearances of '**thumbprinting**'. The colonic wall is inflamed causing severe thickening of the haustral folds, which now appear as 'thumb-shaped' projections into the bowel lumen.

- **Featureless bowel:** Chronic bowel wall thickening causes complete loss of the normal haustral markings. The colon appears smooth walled. In chronic ulcerative colitis the colon can have a classical '**lead pipe**' appearance – the bowel looks like a curvy lead pipe.

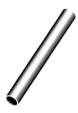

2. **Loss of formed faecal matter in the left-hand side of the colon:** Loss of the normal faecal matter in the left side of the colon indicates that the colon is not functioning properly and is suggestive of bowel wall inflammation.

B

Example 1

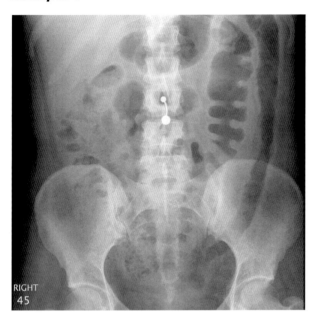
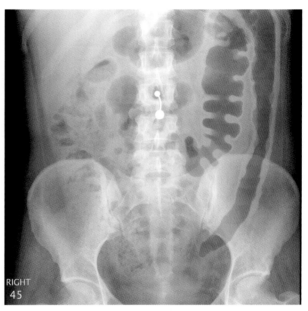

Figure 60: Two identical abdominal radiographs showing colonic bowel wall inflammation. There is thickening of the bowel wall with thickening of the haustral folds in the transverse colon. The descending colon is featureless with loss of the normal haustra. The right radiograph shows the inflamed bowel marked in green and the bowel wall thickening marked in light green. (You can also see an umbilical piercing.)

Example 2

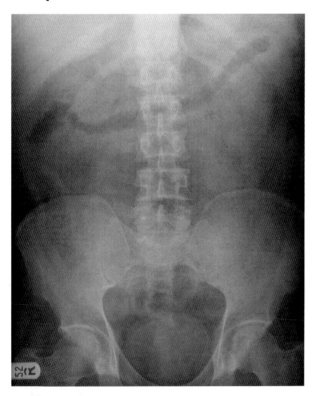
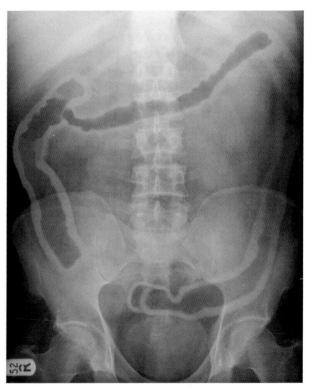

Figure 61: Two identical abdominal radiographs showing bowel wall inflammation throughout the colon. There is thickening of the bowel wall and the colon appears featureless with loss of the normal haustra due to chronic inflammation. This is an example of pancolitis (disease throughout the large intestine). The right radiograph shows the inflamed bowel marked in green and the bowel wall thickening marked in light green.

Example 3

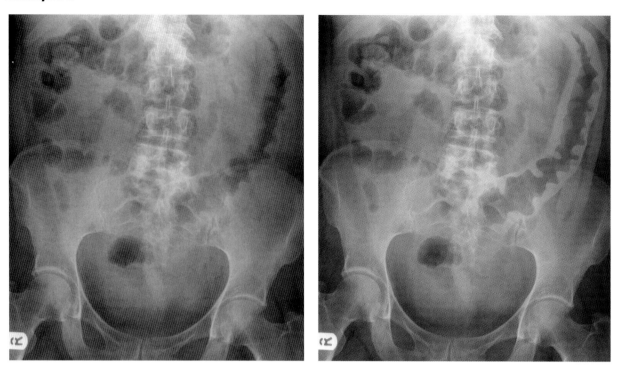

Figure 62: Two identical abdominal radiographs showing colonic bowel wall inflammation. The bowel wall thickening is most easily seen in the transverse colon with severe thickening of the haustral folds giving the appearance of 'thumbprinting'. The right radiograph shows the inflamed bowel marked in green and the bowel wall thickening marked in light green.

Example 4

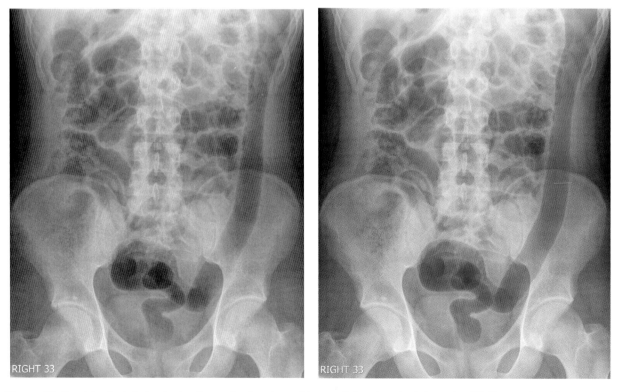

Figure 63: Two identical abdominal radiographs showing evidence of chronic colonic bowel wall inflammation. The rectum, sigmoid and descending colon are featureless with loss of the normal haustra and have a 'lead pipe' appearance. The right radiograph shows the featureless bowel marked in green.

B

Example 5

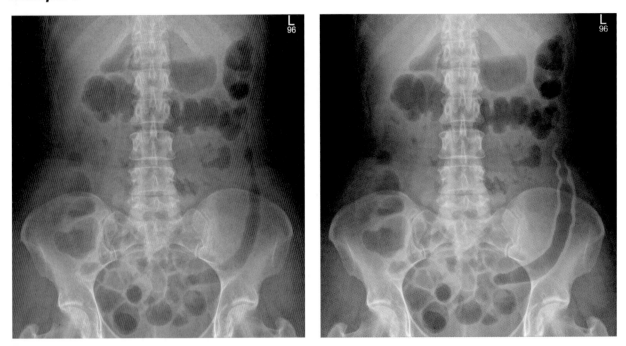

Figure 64: Two identical abdominal radiographs showing colonic bowel wall inflammation. There is slight thickening of the bowel wall, and the descending colon is featureless with loss of the normal haustra giving a 'lead pipe' appearance. The right radiograph shows the featureless bowel marked in green and the bowel wall thickening marked in light green.

Special Case: Toxic Megacolon

Toxic megacolon is an **acute** form of **bowel dilatation** occurring as a complication of **inflammatory bowel disease** (ulcerative colitis or Crohn's) or **infection** (e.g. pseudomembranous colitis from *C. difficile*).

The patient develops rapid dilation of the colon and may show signs of septic shock. If the condition does not improve, it can be **life threatening** and require an emergency colectomy (resection of the diseased colon).

What to look for?

1. **Large bowel dilatation to >6 cm** diameter
2. **Inflammatory pseudopolyps** (mucosal islands): Lobulated opacities in the bowel wall from areas of raised mucosal tissue surrounded by areas of ulceration
3. **Thumbprinting and mucosal oedema** may be present
4. Usually **transverse colon** affected (as in the following example)

Example

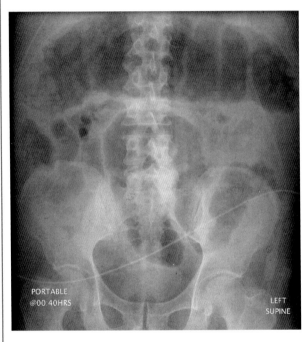
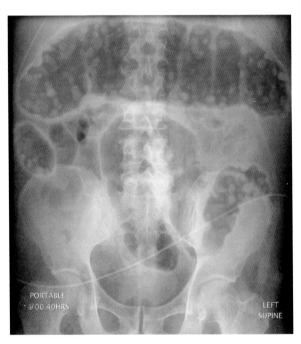

Figure 65: Two identical abdominal radiographs of a patient with toxic megacolon. The transverse colon is dilated to >6 cm diameter. There are multiple small lobulated masses in the lumen in keeping with inflammatory pseudopolyps, and there is evidence of bowel wall thickening. There is also loss of the normal faecal matter within the large bowel. The right radiograph shows the areas of clearly abnormal large bowel marked in green and the thickened bowel wall and inflammatory pseudopolyps marked in light green.

B

Faecal loading

Faecal loading refers to a **large volume of faecal matter** in the **colon** of **any consistency**. Usually this is the result of chronic constipation, although not always, so plain radiographs cannot be used to diagnose constipation.

Hardened faecal matter has a characteristic appearance:

- **Rounded masses**
- **Mottled** or **granular texture** (due to small pockets of gas within the faeces)

Hardened faecal matter within the right side of the colon is highly suggestive of faecal loading as the faecal material here should normally be of fluid consistency.

> **Note:** Constipation is usually a clinical diagnosis without the need for any imaging tests. There is little evidence correlating abdominal X-ray findings with constipation. The only exception is in elderly patients where an abdominal X-ray may be useful to show faecal impaction (*see page 49*).

Example of faecal loading

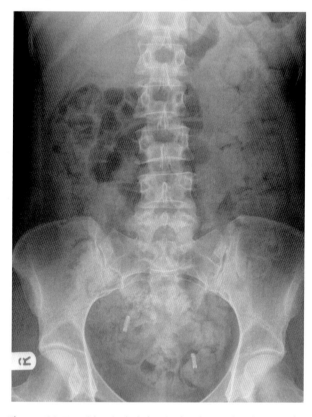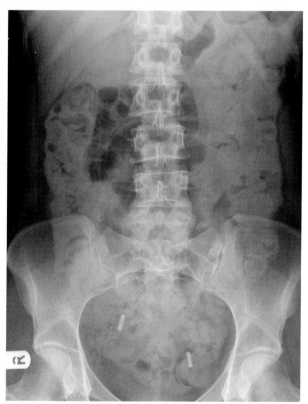

Figure 66: Two identical abdominal radiographs showing faecal loading. There is faecal material throughout the large bowel in keeping with faecal loading. Please note this is not the same as constipation which is a clinical diagnosis. The right radiograph shows the faecal material marked in brown. (You can also see sterilisation clips in the pelvis.)

Faecal impaction

Faecal impaction is more severe than faecal loading and refers to a **solid**, **immobile bulk** of **faeces** that can develop in the **rectum** as a result of chronic constipation. Patients most at risk are the elderly and those who are immobile or institutionalised.

The appearances are usually fairly characteristic with a large (sometimes massive) bulk of faeces in the rectum. In severe cases the impacted faeces can extend into the sigmoid colon and even into the rest of the large bowel.

> **Note:** An abdominal X-ray may be useful to show the extent of faecal impaction, but does not diagnose constipation.

Example of faecal impaction

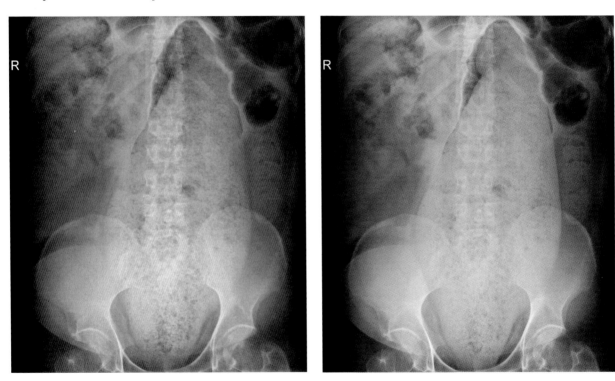

Figure 67: Two identical abdominal radiographs showing faecal impaction. There is a huge volume of faecal material extending from the pelvis to the left upper quadrant in keeping with a huge faecal impaction causing massive distension of the rectum. The right radiograph shows the faecal material marked in brown.

Gallstones in the gallbladder (cholelithiasis)

Cholelithiasis is the presence of **gallstones** in the **gallbladder**.

Approximately 10% of the population have gallstones; however, only around 15% of gallstones contain enough calcium to be visible on a plain radiograph. Therefore some gallstones will be clearly visible, and some will only just be visible and the majority will be invisible due to lack of calcium content.

If gallstones are visible, they will be seen projected over the **right upper quadrant** along the lower border of the liver. Their appearances can be very variable:

- May be **large or small**
- May be **single or multiple**
- May have a **radiopaque (dense) outline** with a **lucent centre**
- May have a **polygonal shape** (smooth flat surfaces) due to stones abutting one another
- May have a **laminated** (concentric rings) appearance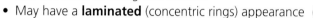

> **Note:** Ultrasound of the abdomen is the investigation of choice for suspected gallstones. A plain abdominal radiograph should not be performed as the majority of gallstones comprise cholesterol and bile pigments which are not radiopaque and do not show up on a plain radiograph. Nevertheless, gallstones are an important incidental finding to report if seen on an abdominal radiograph.

Example 1

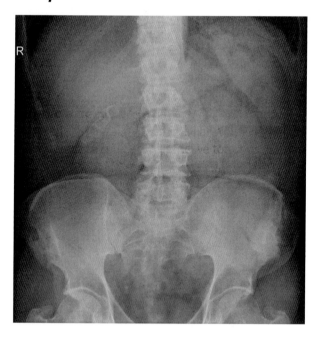 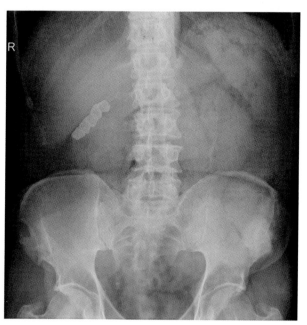

Figure 68: Two identical abdominal radiographs showing calcified gallstones projected over the right upper quadrant. In this example the gallstones are polygonal in shape and have a radiopaque outline with a lucent centre. The right radiograph shows the gallstones marked in yellow.

Example 2

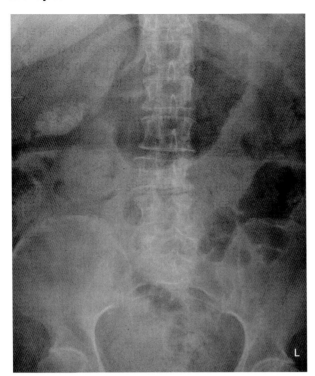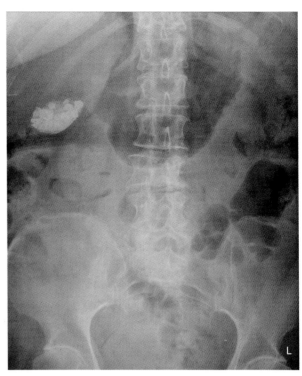

Figure 69: Two identical abdominal radiographs of the abdomen showing calcified gallstones projected over the right upper quadrant. In this example there are many gallstones of varying size. They are polygonal in shape and have a radiopaque outline with a lucent centre. The gallstones are seen to clearly outline the lower border of the gallbladder. The right radiograph shows the gallstones marked in yellow.

Special Cases: Milk of Calcium or 'Limey' Bile

A rare condition in which the gallbladder contains a **dense fluid** usually containing **calcium carbonate**. This allows it to be visualised on an abdominal radiograph.

This condition is always associated with gallstones (which may or may not be visible).

It gives the following appearances:

- **Radiopaque gallbladder lumen**
- **Gallstones may be seen outlined by the bile**

Example

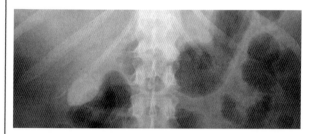 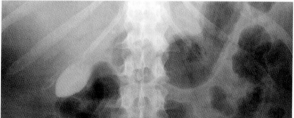

Figure 70: Two identical radiographs of the upper abdomen showing milk of calcium or 'limey' bile. There is a rounded gallbladder-shaped density projected over the right upper quadrant. If you look carefully you can see a few circular gallstones outlined at the superior aspect of the gallbladder. The right radiograph shows the milk of calcium or 'limey' bile marked in yellow.

Porcelain gallbladder

A porcelain gallbladder refers to a gallbladder with **heavily calcified walls**. It is associated with an increased risk of developing **gallbladder malignancy**, therefore a cholecystectomy is usually recommended. The name comes from its bluish colour (at time of surgery) and brittle nature (like porcelain).

Radiological appearance:

- **Rim of calcification outlining the gallbladder:** The wall of the gallbladder is calcified with the edge appearing more dense than the centre

Example

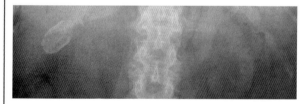 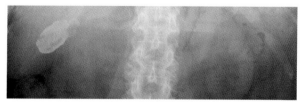

Figure 71: Two identical radiographs of the upper abdomen showing a porcelain gallbladder. There is a curvilinear gallbladder-shaped area of calcification projected over the right upper quadrant. The right radiograph shows the porcelain gallbladder marked in yellow.

Renal stones (urolithiasis)

Renal stones, renal calculi, kidney stones and urolithiasis all refer to stone formation within the renal tract. A renal stone is termed a **calculus** (*calculi (pl)*). It is a concentration of inorganic material, originating in the renal pelvis or calyces.

Sometimes renal calculi migrate into the ureter and are then termed **ureteric calculi**. This may lead to renal outflow obstruction and renal colic.

Most renal stones (**90%**) contain enough calcium to be visible on a plain radiograph, although some such as uric acid stones and pure matrix stones are radiolucent and are not visualised.

Radiological signs:
- **Calcific density projected over the kidney:** Look carefully over the region of the kidneys for any small calcific densities.
- **Calcific density projected over the course of the ureter:** The ureter runs from the medial aspect of the kidney and inferiorly along the tips of the transverse processes. Look carefully over the course of the ureter for any small calcific densities, which may appear very subtle.
- **'Staghorn' calculus:** Sometimes a large renal stone can fill and take the shape of all or part of the renal pelvis and calyces to give a classical 'staghorn' shape (see Figures 73 and 74).

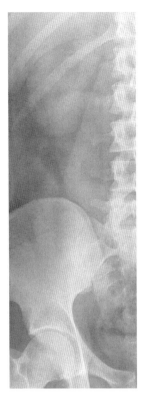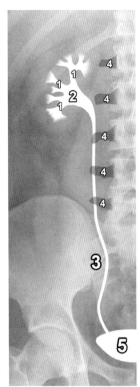

Figure 72: Two identical radiographs of the right side of the abdomen with the path of the urinary tract marked in white. A calculus may be found at any point along the tract. Renal calculi will be seen in the region of the calyces (1) or renal pelvis (2). Ureteric calculi are seen along the line of the ureter (3) which runs along the line of the transverse processes (4). Bladder calculi will be seen in the region of the urinary bladder (5).

If renal calculi are suspected clinically, then the most appropriate imaging test is a low-dose CT scan of the kidneys, ureters and bladder (CT KUB). A CT KUB is far more sensitive and specific than a plain radiograph for detecting the presence of renal calculi. Plain radiographs may be useful in the follow-up of known moderate to large-sized renal calculi.

Example 1

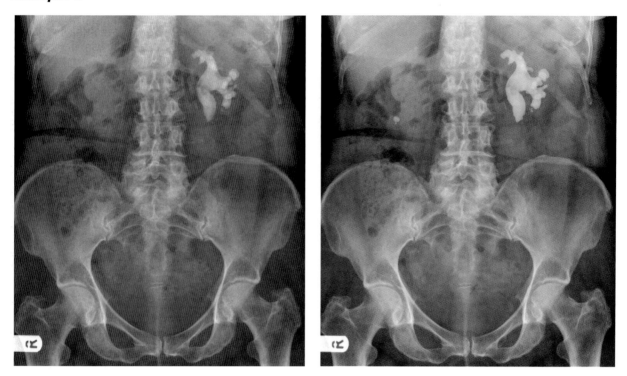

Figure 73: Two identical abdominal radiographs showing a left staghorn calculus and right-sided renal calculi. There is a large staghorn-shaped calcific density seen projected over the left kidney and two smaller calcific densities are noted projected over the right kidney. The right radiograph shows the left staghorn calculus and right renal calculi marked in yellow.

Example 2

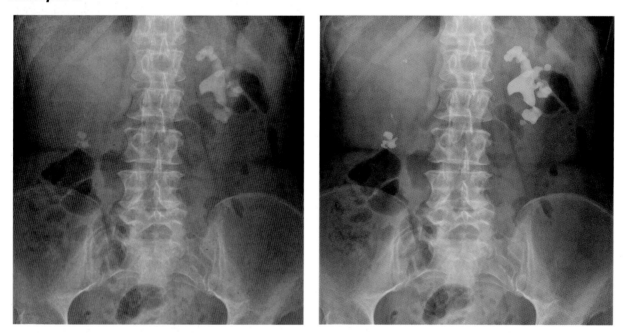

Figure 74: Two identical abdominal radiographs showing a left staghorn calculus and right-sided renal calculi. There is a large staghorn-shaped calcific density projected over the left kidney and a few smaller calcific densities are noted projected over the right kidney. The right radiograph shows the left staghorn calculus and right renal calculi marked in yellow.

Example 3

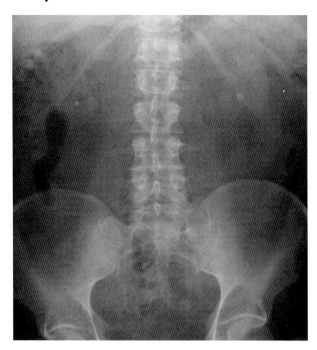 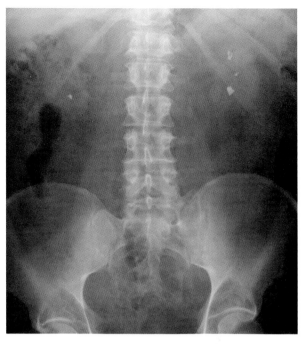

Figure 75: Two identical abdominal radiographs showing bilateral renal calculi. There are a few small calcific densities projected over the left kidney and a small calcific density is projected over the lower pole of the right kidney in keeping with renal calculi. The right radiograph shows the renal calculi marked in yellow.

Example 4

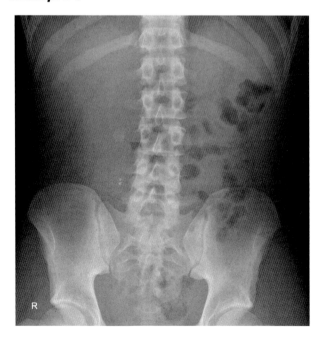 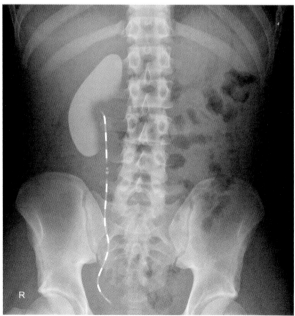

Figure 76: Two identical abdominal radiographs showing ureteric calculi. There are two small calcific densities projected to the right of the lumbar spine. These are most likely in keeping with ureteric calculi as they are projected over the line of the right ureter and are too small to be calcified lymph nodes. The right radiograph shows the ureteric calculi marked in yellow, the position of the right kidney marked in white and the line of the right ureter marked with a white dashed line.

Bladder stones

A bladder stone (or **bladder calculus**) refers to the formation of a dense stone within the urinary bladder. The main causes are as follows:

1. **Urinary stasis (most common)**
   - Bladder outlet obstruction, for example from enlarged prostate
   - Bladder diverticulum
   - Neurogenic bladder, for example spinal cord injury/paralysis
2. **Urinary infections**
3. **Migrated renal calculus**
4. **Foreign material left in place**
   - Long-term urinary catheterisation

 They appear as rounded or oval-shaped opacities projected over the lower pelvis near the midline. They are often large and may be multiple. Some may have a **laminated** (concentric rings) appearance.

> **Note:** Phleboliths are commonly seen within the pelvis, so do not mistake these for bladder calculi. They are often much smaller and more numerous than bladder calculi (*see page 63*).

Example 1

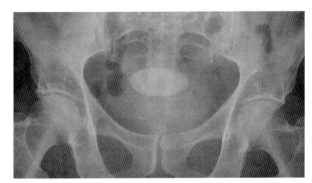 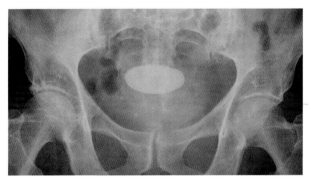

Figure 77: Two identical abdominal radiographs showing a bladder calculus. There is a large, midline, oval-shaped opacity projected over the lower pelvis. The right radiograph shows the bladder calculus marked in yellow.

Example 2

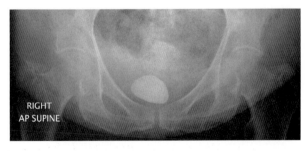 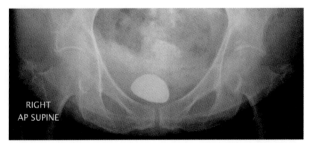

Figure 78: Two identical abdominal radiographs showing a bladder calculus. There is a large, roughly midline, oval-shaped opacity projected over the lower pelvis. If you look carefully at the outer edge, there is the impression of a thin dense line in keeping with a slight laminated appearance. The right radiograph shows the bladder calculus marked in yellow.

Nephrocalcinosis

Nephrocalcinosis refers to abnormal deposition of **calcium** in the **kidney parenchyma**. It can affect the cortex (cortical nephrocalcinosis) or medulla (medullary nephrocalcinosis), but the **medulla** is far more commonly affected. It is usually associated with **metabolic** disorders.

Main causes include the following:

1. Hyperparathyroidism
2. Medullary sponge kidney
3. Renal tubular acidosis

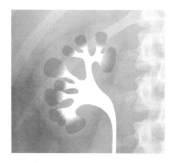

The radiographic appearances are quite distinctive:

- Calcium deposition is usually **generalised** rather than local.
- Often the calcification is seen in little **clusters**. These clusters correspond to the **medullary pyramids** (see Figure 79).

Figure 79: The right kidney with the pelvicalyceal system marked in white. The medullary pyramids are marked in brown.

Example 1

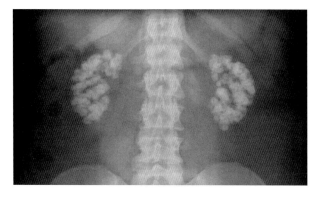

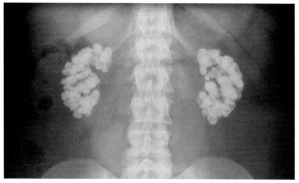

Figure 80: Two identical abdominal radiographs showing medullary nephrocalcinosis. There are multiple patchy calcifications throughout both kidneys. If you look carefully, it appears as if the renal pelvis and calyces are spared indicating that the calcification is affecting the renal parenchyma. The right radiograph shows the nephrocalcinosis marked in yellow.

Example 2

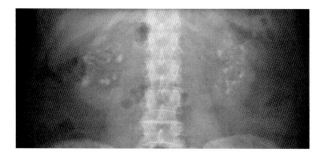

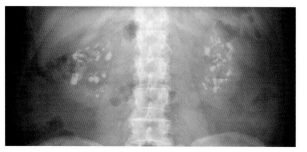

Figure 81: Two identical abdominal radiographs showing medullary nephrocalcinosis. There are multiple patchy calcifications throughout both kidneys. The right radiograph shows the nephrocalcinosis marked in yellow.

Pancreatic calcification

Pancreatic calcification is the formation of **small foci of calcification** within the **pancreas**. It is most commonly a sign of **chronic pancreatitis**. The most common underlying cause is **alcohol abuse**.

> **Note:** The pancreas is a retroperitoneal structure, which crosses the midline and in normal patients is not visualised on an abdominal radiograph.

The radiographic appearance is of **irregular clusters** or **foci** of calcification crossing the **midline** in the **mid-abdomen**. If the calcification is extensive, then it will be seen to take the rough shape of the pancreas.

Example 1

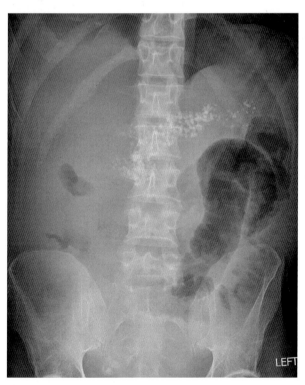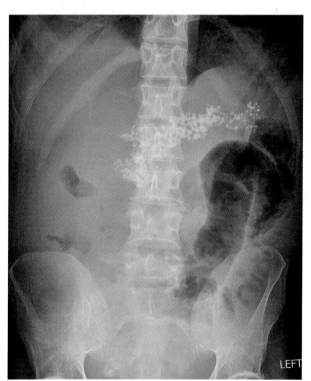

Figure 82: Two identical abdominal radiographs showing pancreatic calcification. There are multiple irregular foci of calcification projected over the midline in the rough shape of the pancreas. The right radiograph shows the pancreatic calcifications marked in yellow.

Example 2

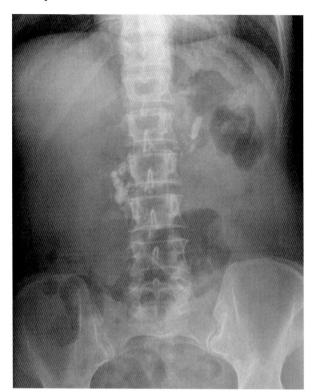
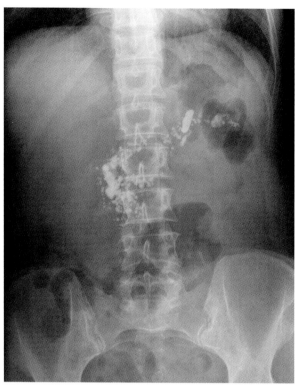

Figure 83: Two identical abdominal radiographs showing pancreatic calcification. There are multiple irregular foci of calcification projected over the midline in the rough shape of the pancreas. The right radiograph shows the pancreatic calcifications marked in yellow.

Adrenal calcification

Adrenal calcification is uncommon and usually an incidental finding. It is often associated with previous **adrenal haemorrhage** or **tuberculosis (TB)**.

The radiographic appearance is of a **triangular**-shaped area of **irregular** calcification projected in the region of the upper pole of the kidney.

Example

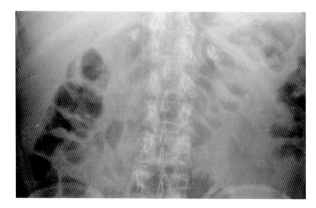
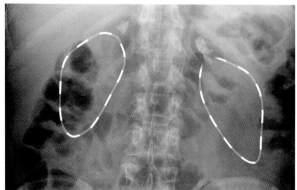

Figure 84: Two identical abdominal radiographs showing bilateral adrenal gland calcification. There are bilateral areas of irregular calcification projected either side of the midline at the level of the upper pole of the kidneys. The right radiograph shows the adrenal gland calcification marked in yellow and the approximate position of the kidneys (not seen clearly) marked with a white dashed line.

Abdominal aortic aneurysm (AAA) calcification

An AAA, pronounced 'triple-a', is **abnormal dilatation** of the abdominal aorta to **>3 cm diameter**. Normally the aorta should measure <2.5 cm in diameter.

Most aneurysms are asymptomatic. The incidence of AAA is 5–10%, and they tend to progressively enlarge over time. The larger the AAA becomes, the higher the risk of rupture. Rupture of an AAA is associated with a very high mortality rate (>80%).

When the AAA grows to >5.5 cm the risk of aneurysm rupture outweighs the risk of operative management, and treatment is recommended either by open surgery or endovascular aneurysm repair (EVAR).

AAAs are only occasionally seen on an abdominal radiograph. When seen, they have the following appearances:

- An AAA will only be visualised on an abdominal radiograph if there is **calcification** in the **wall** of the **aorta**. Wall calcification appears as white lines seen projected over the lower abdomen, outlining the wall of the aorta.
- **Both** sides of the aortic wall must be visualised to diagnose an AAA. If only one side of the wall of the aorta is seen bulging to the left or right of the spine then you cannot diagnose an AAA as the aorta may be ectatic (tortuous) without being aneurysmal.
- **Most** (>90%) **are infra-renal** (below the origin of the renal arteries)

> **Note:** If found incidentally on an abdominal radiograph, a CT scan is usually recommended to properly assess the size of the AAA and, if necessary, plan for surgery.

Example 1

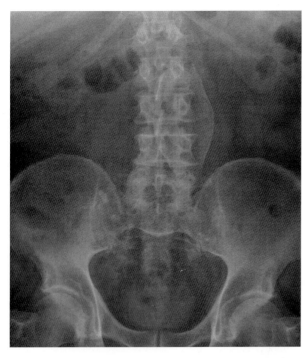 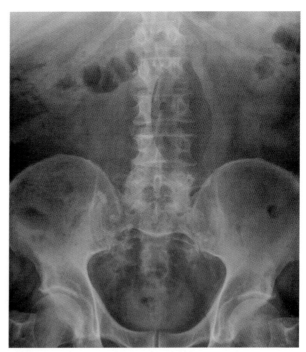

Figure 85: Two identical abdominal radiographs showing AAA calcification. There is a large dilated vascular structure in the midline with wall calcification seen. The left wall is clearly seen; however, the right wall is more difficult to make out as it is projected over the lumbar spine. It measures over 3 cm in diameter. The right radiograph shows the AAA marked in red.

Example 2

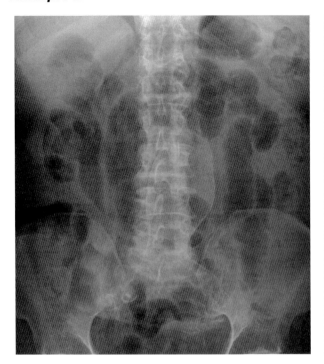 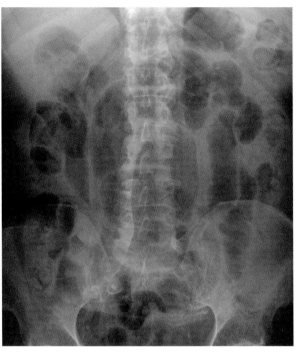

Figure 86: Two identical abdominal radiographs showing AAA calcification. There is a large dilated vascular structure in the midline with wall calcification seen. The left wall is clearly seen; however, the right wall is more difficult to make out as it is projected over the lumbar spine. It measures over 3 cm in diameter. The right radiograph shows the AAA marked in red.

Example 3

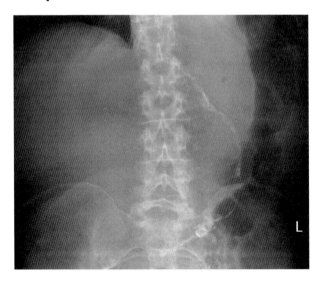 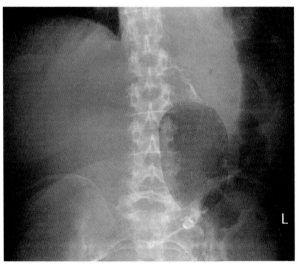

Figure 87: Two identical abdominal radiographs showing AAA calcification. There is a large dilated vascular structure in the midline with wall calcification seen. The left wall is clearly seen; however, the right wall is more difficult to make out as it is projected over the lumbar spine. It measures over 3 cm in diameter. The right radiograph shows the AAA marked in red.

Fetus

A fetus refers to the developing human from the embryonic stage (11 weeks gestation) to birth. Seeing a fetus on an abdominal radiograph is very rare as **ionising radiation should be avoided in pregnancy** due to the slight increased risk of fetal teratogenesis and carcinogenesis. If imaging is required, then an alternative investigation such as an ultrasound scan is usually advised.

On an abdominal radiograph the fetus is visualised once the skeleton starts to calcify. Look for a '**skeleton within the abdomen**'. Often a **large circular opacity** (fetal head) and a **linear array of smaller opacities** (fetal spine) are identifiable.

Example

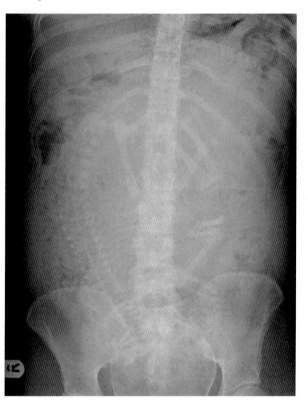 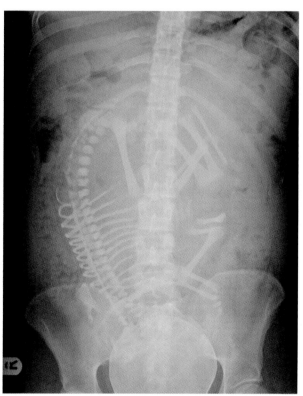

Figure 88: Two identical abdominal radiographs showing a fetus in situ. The spine of the fetus can be seen to the right of the midline, lower limbs in the upper abdomen, upper limbs in the centre of the abdomen and the skull in the pelvis. This fetus is large and nearly term. The right radiograph shows the skeleton of the fetus marked in yellow.

Note on radiation risk: All female patients between the ages of 12 and 55 years should be asked if there is a possibility that they are pregnant before being exposed to ionising radiation. If a female patient undergoing an abdominal or pelvic radiograph has a missed period, the patient should be considered pregnant until proved otherwise. The absolute increased radiation risk to the fetus from an abdominal radiograph is tiny. To put this in perspective, it is good to compare the fetal dose from an abdominal radiograph to the natural background radiation dose a fetus will receive over 9 months gestation. Using this comparison, the dose from an abdominal radiograph is equivalent to approximately 4 months background radiation. For more information on reducing radiation risk, see section on Hazards and Precautions (*see page 3*)

Calcified structures of little clinical significance

There are many structures that can calcify on a normal abdominal radiograph. It is important to be aware of these so that they do not cause diagnostic confusion.

Calcified costal cartilage

In many patients, the costal cartilage is not calcified and therefore not visualised (Example 1).

In some patients however, the costal cartilage is calcified (Example 2), often appearing patchy and more dense than the ribs. It is typically seen as a continuation of the ribs, curving superiorly and medially.

Although this appearance is more common with age, young patients may also have cartilage calcification. This is a normal finding.

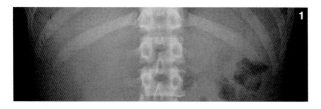
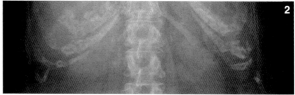
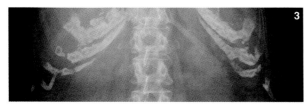

Figure 89: The top radiograph (1) shows a patient without costal cartilage calcification. The middle radiograph (2) shows a patient with costal cartilage calcification. The bottom radiograph (3) shows the calcification marked in yellow.

Phleboliths ('vein stones')

Phleboliths are small focal calcifications within veins. They are commonly seen within the pelvis and usually have no clinical significance.

They appear as small, rounded opacities, sometimes with a lucent centre. There may be just one or two, or sometimes there are many scattered throughout the pelvis.

It is important to recognise phleboliths, so you do not incorrectly mistake them for renal calculi. If ureteric or bladder calculi are suspected, then an alternative investigation such as an unenhanced CT scan is more sensitive and specific.

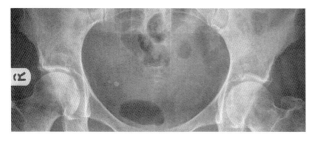
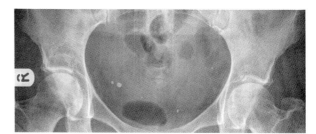
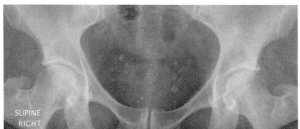
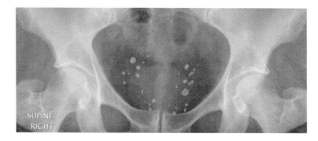

Figure 90: Two pairs of identical abdominal radiographs showing phleboliths in the pelvis. They are of calcific density and a few show the classical lucent centre. The phleboliths are marked in yellow.

Calcified mesenteric lymph nodes

Calcified mesenteric lymph nodes are a common incidental finding. They are lymph nodes normally found in the bowel mesentery, which have become calcified, usually secondary to a previous granulomatous infection such as TB. They are commonly seen in elderly patients.

They appear as oval-shaped, mottled areas of calcification, usually 5–15 mm in size, often seen in the right lower quadrant or central abdomen. Normally they appear in clusters of two or more.

> **Note:** The mottled appearance and location usually distinguishes calcified lymph nodes from renal calculi; however if projected over the kidney or path of the ureter, it can be difficult to exclude a renal calculus. A characteristic feature of calcified mesenteric lymph nodes is that they change position between different radiographs (as the bowel mesentery is quite mobile within the peritoneal cavity), therefore comparison with previous radiographs can often help with their identification.

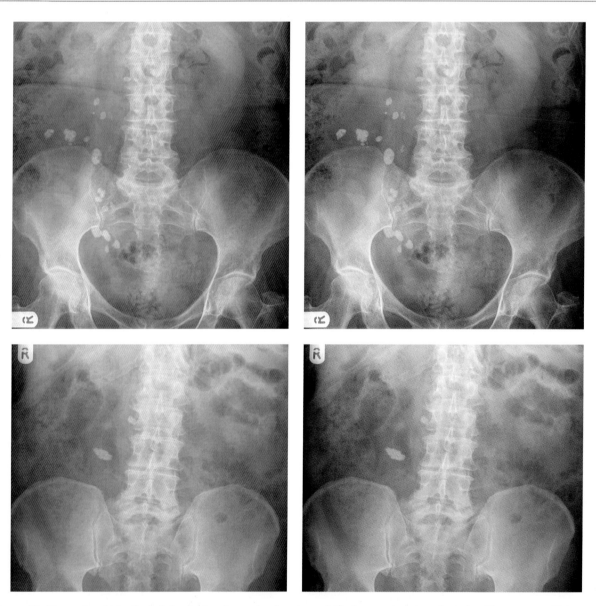

Figure 91: Two pairs of identical abdominal radiographs showing calcified mesenteric lymph nodes. There are multiple oval-shaped areas of mottled calcification projected over the right lower quadrant/central abdomen. The calcified lymph nodes are marked in yellow.

Calcified uterine fibroids

Uterine fibroids (leiomyomas) are benign tumours of myometrial origin. Longstanding fibroids may calcify and appear on an abdominal radiograph as rounded calcified structures within the pelvis with 'splatter'-like calcification. They may appear similar to bladder calculi. Often these are incidental findings.

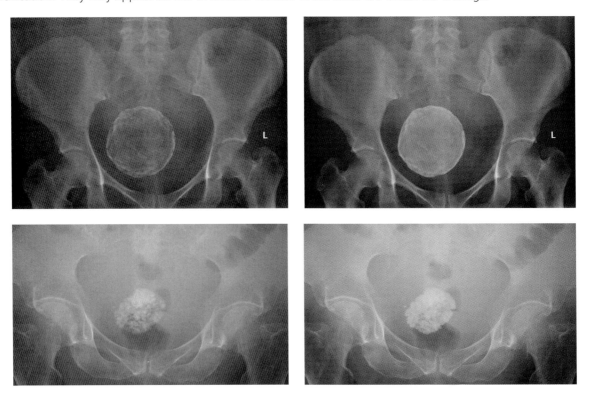

Figure 92: Two pairs of identical abdominal radiographs showing calcified uterine fibroids. There are rounded areas of calcification projected over the pelvis with irregular areas of calcification within. The calcified uterine fibroids are marked in yellow.

Prostate calcification

Calcification of the prostate gland may occur in older men. It appears as fine or coarse calcification in the lower pelvis, just below the position of the urinary bladder. Often only part of the gland is calcified. It is an incidental finding.

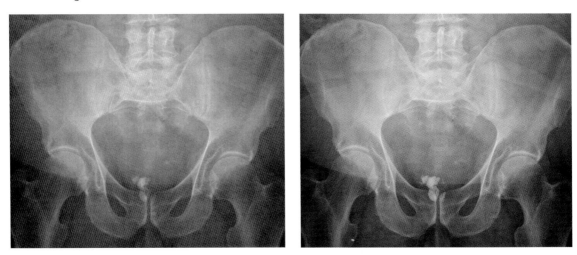

Figure 93: Two identical abdominal radiographs showing calcification of the prostate gland. There is irregular calcification projected over the lower pelvis just below the position of the urinary bladder. The right radiograph shows the prostate gland calcification marked in yellow.

Abdominal aortic calcification (normal calibre)

In elderly and diabetic patients the wall of the aorta (and other major arteries) may calcify. This is indicative of atheromatous processes in the wall of the vessel. Look for linear areas of calcification projected over the midline.

> **Note:** In elderly patients the abdominal aorta may take a tortuous course.

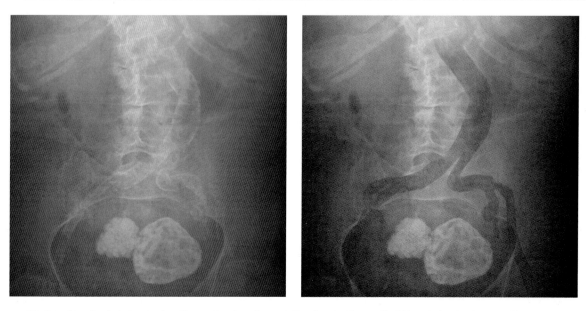

Figure 94: Two identical abdominal radiographs showing calcification in the wall of the abdominal aorta. There are areas of linear calcification outlining the abdominal aorta, common iliac arteries, external iliac arteries and proximal internal iliac arteries. The aorta is less than 2.5 cm in diameter; therefore this is not an abdominal aortic aneurysm. The right radiograph shows the calcified vascular structures marked in red. (You can also see two calcified uterine fibroids and costal cartilage calcification.)

Splenic artery calcification

The splenic artery is another vascular structure that is commonly calcified. It is seen projected over the left upper quadrant and has a distinctive tortuous 'Chinese Dragon'-like appearance.

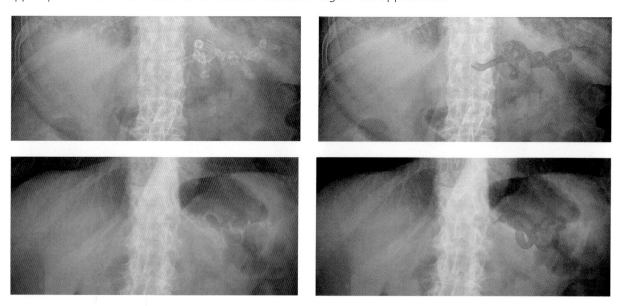

Figure 95: Two pairs of identical abdominal radiographs showing calcification in the wall of the splenic artery. There are areas of linear calcification projected over the left upper quadrant with a tortuous 'Chinese Dragon'-like appearance outlining the splenic artery. The right radiograph shows the calcified splenic artery marked in red.

Pelvic fractures – 3 Polo rings test

If the pelvis is included on the radiograph it is important to check for pelvic fractures. The best way to look for fractures is to consider the pelvis to be comprised of three rings:

1. **Pelvic ring:** The paired ilium, ischium and pubic bones along with the sacrum are held together by tough ligaments to form a large pelvic ring.
2. **Ring of bone surrounding the right obturator foramen**
3. **Ring of bone surrounding the left obturator foramen**

Now imagine these rings act like three large **Polo mints**. It is impossible to break a Polo mint in one place – it must break in at least two places. Therefore if you see a fracture in one part of the ring, look for the second fracture (or disruption of the pubic symphysis or sacroiliac joints). It is almost impossible to have a significant fracture in one place and not another.

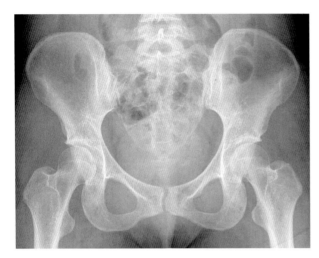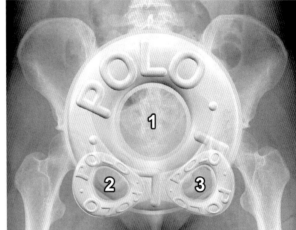

Figure 96: Two identical radiographs of a normal pelvis showing the 3 Polo rings. The right radiograph shows the pelvic ring (1), ring of bone surrounding the right obturator foramen (2) and ring of bone surrounding the left obturator foramen (3) marked with Polo rings.

Example

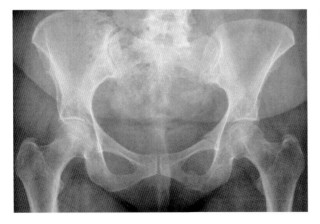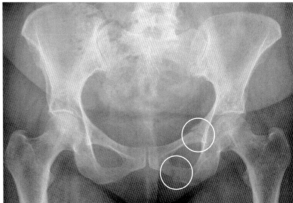

Figure 97: Two identical pelvic radiographs showing fractures of the superior and inferior pubic rami, and left iliac bone. The ring of bone surrounding the left obturator foramen has fractured in two places like a Polo ring. These two fractures have caused disruption of the larger pelvic ring and, although not seen on this radiograph, a further break in the larger pelvic ring is likely. The right radiograph shows the fractures marked with a white circle.

Sclerotic and lucent bone lesions

These can occur anywhere within the skeleton (pelvis, spine, etc).

Sclerotic lesion: Abnormal area of **increased density** (whiter) within the bone. There are many causes for sclerotic bone lesions including malignancy. **Prostate metastases** are a common cause of multiple sclerotic lesions within the pelvis or spine.

Lucent lesion: Abnormal area of **reduced density** (blacker) within the bone. Again there is a wide differential diagnosis for a lucent lesion including malignancy.

> **Note:** If there is any doubt as to the likely diagnosis, then discussion with a radiologist is advised.

Example of a sclerotic bone lesion

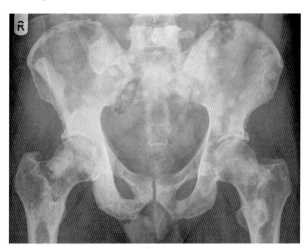 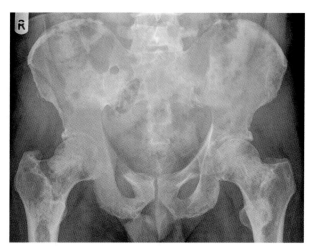

Figure 98: Two pairs of identical radiographs showing multiple sclerotic bone lesions. There are multiple areas of increased density throughout the pelvis. In this elderly male patient the most likely cause is prostate metastasis. The right radiograph shows the sclerotic lesions marked in red.

Example of a lucent bone lesion

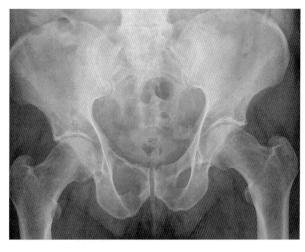 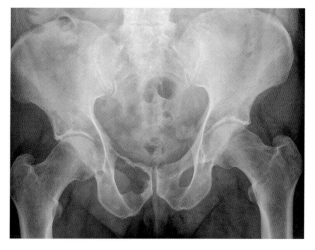

Figure 99: Two pairs of identical radiographs showing a lucent bone lesion. If you compare the left and right sides, you can see an ill-defined area of lucency in the right pubic bone, with loss of the normal dense bone appearance. In this case the lucent lesion was a metastasis. The right radiograph shows the lucent lesion marked in red.

Spine pathology

It is important to remember to look carefully at the spine on an abdominal radiograph.

> **What to look for?**
> - **Vertebral body height:** The vertebral body heights should be roughly the same. Look for a vertebral body which appears shorter in height than the others above and below it. Loss of height may indicate a vertebral compression fracture. It is not usually possible to tell whether a fracture is acute or chronic using a plain radiograph.

Examples

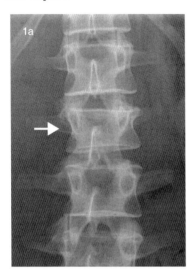 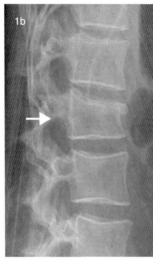 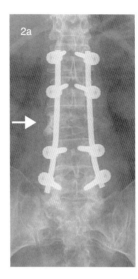 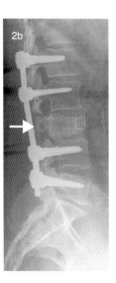

Figure 100: (1a) AP and (1b) lateral radiographs of the lumbar spine in the same patient showing an example of a wedge compression fracture of the L2 vertebral body. Note how there is loss of height of the L2 vertebral body (white arrow) when compared to the vertebrae above and below. (2a) AP and (2b) lateral radiographs of the lumbar spine in the same patient showing an example of a compression fracture of the L3 vertebral body. Note how there is loss of height of the L3 vertebral body (white arrow) when compared to the vertebrae above and below. There is also spinal metal work in situ providing mechanical support to the lumbar spine either side of the fracture.

> - **Alignment:** The spine should look straight. If the spine is curved to the left or right side, then the patient may have scoliosis.

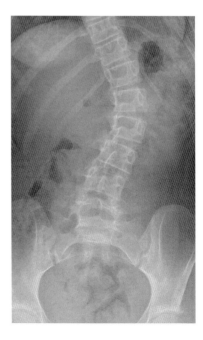

Figure 101: A radiograph of a patient with thoraco-lumbar scoliosis. The thoraco-lumbar spine is curved with concavity to the right.

- **Pedicles:** Ensure you can see both the left and right pedicle on all of the visualised vertebrae. Loss of visualisation of a pedicle may indicate a destructive bone lesion (e.g. a metastasis) causing erosion and loss of visualisation of the pedicle. An abnormally dense pedicle may indicate a sclerotic bone lesion (e.g. a metastasis).

Figure 102: Diagram of a vertebra as seen from above with both left and right pedicles marked in yellow.

Example

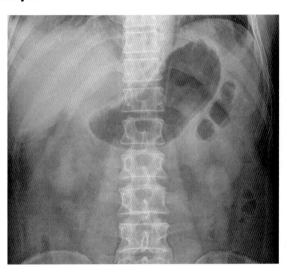
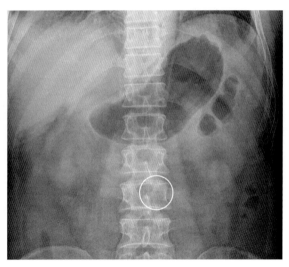

Figure 103: Two identical abdominal radiographs showing absence of the left L3 pedicle due to destruction by a spinal metastasis. The normal dense oval shape of the left pedicle of L3 is no longer visualised. The right radiograph shows the position of the missing pedicle shown with a white circle.

- **'Bamboo spine':** Seen in patients with **ankylosing spondylitis**. Patients have ossification of the interspinous and supraspinous ligaments, and marginal syndesmophytes causing fusion (ankylosis) of the vertebrae. The resulting appearance is referred to as a 'bamboo spine'.

Example

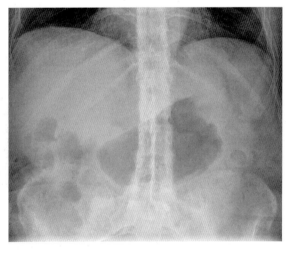
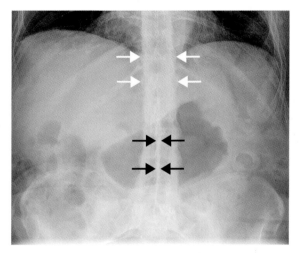

Figure 104: Two identical abdominal radiographs showing a 'bamboo spine' in a patient with ankylosing spondylitis. There is a dense vertical line in the midline caused by ossification of the interspinous and supraspinous ligaments (black arrows). There is fusion (ankylosis) of the vertebrae by marginal syndesmophytes (white arrows). This gives the overall appearance of a spine that looks a bit like a bamboo stick. The right radiograph shows the 'Bamboo spine' marked in yellow.

Solid organ enlargement

Solid organ enlargement may be caused by an increase in the overall size of one of the **solid organs** or by a **large tumour** in the abdomen. It is usually an incidental finding on an abdominal radiograph as the initial investigation of choice for an abdominal mass is usually an ultrasound scan. An abdominal X-ray can raise the possibility of solid organ enlargement, but cannot characterise it. Common causes of solid organ enlargement are as follows:

- Solid organ:
  - **Hepatomegaly** (enlargement of the liver)
    - **Riedel's lobe:** Inferior, tongue-like projection of the right lobe of the liver. A normal anatomical variant seen in approximately 17% of the population.
  - **Splenomegaly** (enlargement of the spleen)
- Tumour:
  - **Renal mass** (e.g. large renal cyst or renal malignancy)
  - **Pelvic mass** (e.g. large ovarian cyst or ovarian malignancy)

Radiological signs:
- Large soft tissue density (light grey) mass
- Loops of bowel often displaced by the mass
- Location often gives a clue as to the origin:
  - right upper quadrant: liver, right kidney
  - left upper quadrant: spleen, left kidney, fluid filled stomach
  - lower abdomen: ovaries, uterus, distended urinary bladder

Example 1

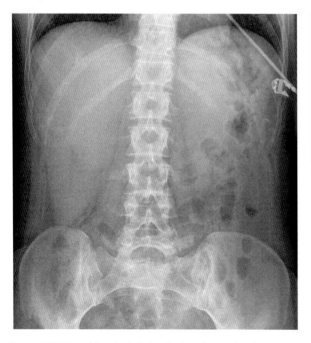 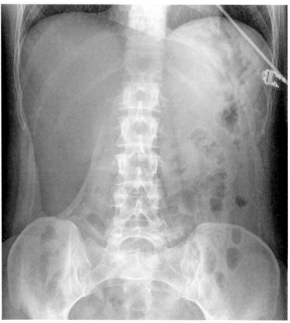

Figure 105: Two identical abdominal radiographs showing a Riedel's lobe (normal variant). The right lobe of the liver is enlarged and extends inferiorly. The right radiograph shows the enlarged liver marked in purple. (You can also see an ECG lead in the left upper quadrant).

D

Example 2

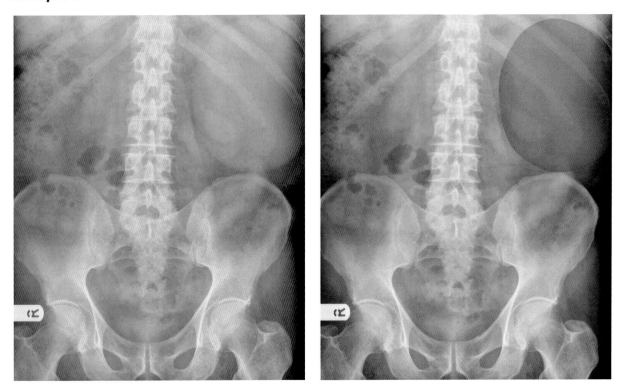

Figure 106: Two identical abdominal radiographs showing a large soft tissue mass in the left lumbar region. There is a rounded soft tissue density in the region of the left kidney. In this case the underlying cause was a large renal cyst. The right radiograph shows the soft tissue mass marked in red.

Example 3

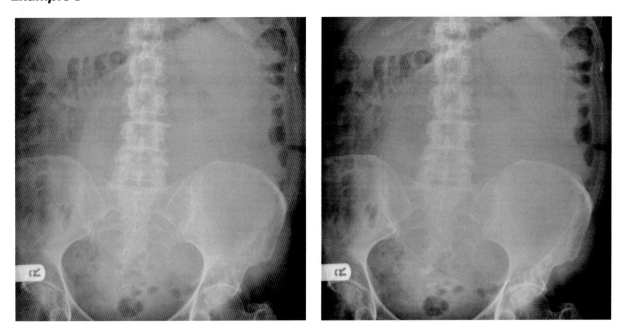

Figure 107: Two identical abdominal radiographs showing a large soft tissue mass in the pelvis/central abdomen. There is a large soft tissue density arising from the pelvis and extending into the left upper quadrant. It is displacing the surrounding loops of bowel to the edge of the radiograph. In this case the underlying cause was a large ovarian cyst. The right radiograph shows the large pelvic/central abdominal mass marked in pink.

Medical and surgical objects (iatrogenic)

It is common to see metallic objects, tubes and other surgically placed objects in the abdomen. Identifying these is important and may help you figure out what is wrong with the patient.

Surgical clips/staples/sutures

Surgical clips, staples and anastomoses are common findings on abdominal radiographs. It is important to recognise the differences between them.

Examples of cholecystectomy (removal of the gallbladder) clips

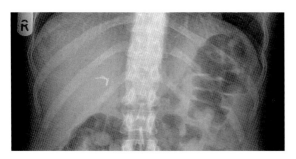

Figure 108: Two different radiographs showing metallic cholecystectomy clips projected over the right upper quadrant in the region of the gallbladder. This is a very common finding as cholecystectomy is a common operation. Usually there are three clips, although there may be more.

Examples of female sterilisation clips

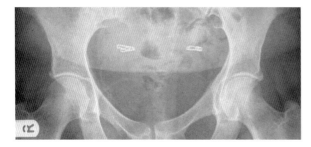

Figure 109: Two different radiographs showing sterilisation clips projected over the pelvis. They have a distinctive appearance and there are usually one or two clips seen bilaterally (for each of the fallopian tubes). Often over time these clips migrate and can be seen elsewhere in the abdomen (e.g. under the liver) – this is not a problem.

Example of hepatectomy clips

Example of surgical staples

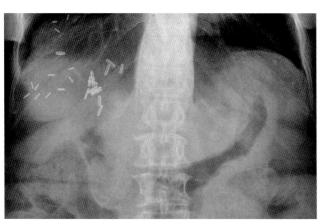

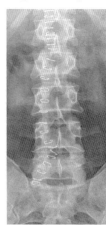

Figure 110: A radiograph showing numerous surgical clips projected over the right upper quadrant. This appearance is typical for previous liver resection surgery.

Figure 111: A radiograph showing surgical staples projected over the midline from a recent midline laparotomy.

E

Example of hernia clips

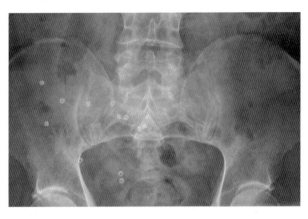
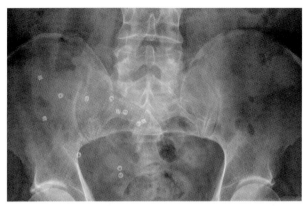

Figure 112: Two identical radiographs showing evidence of a right inguinal hernia repair. There are multiple helical coil fasteners projected over the right iliac fossa. The appearance of these small coils is characteristic and indicates the site of a previous hernia repair. The coils fasten a surgical mesh to the inside of the abdominal wall to cover any areas of weakness and prevent a hernia. The mesh is not normally visualised on an abdominal radiograph. The right radiograph shows the rough position of the hernia mesh repair marked in orange.

Examples of surgical bowel anastomoses

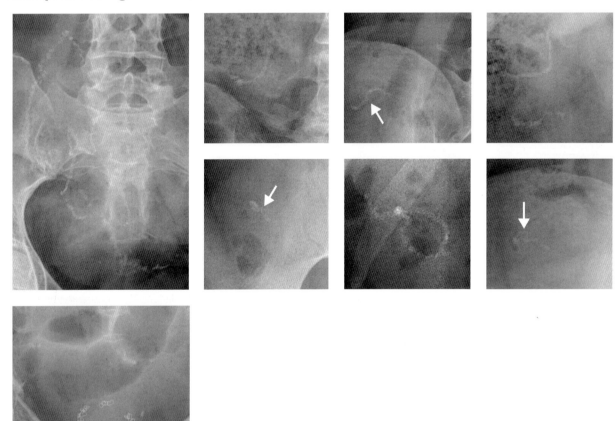

Figure 113: Eight different radiographs of bowel anastomoses. They may be tricky to visualise as they are very small and not particularly dense. They appear as a curly line of multiple tiny clips and indicate the site of a bowel anastomosis. In a few of the radiographs the bowel anastomoses are very difficult to visualise so are marked with white arrows.

E

Urinary catheter

A urinary catheter is a **hollow flexible tube** inserted into the urinary bladder via the urethra to drain urine from the bladder. They are common and easy to recognise due to their classical position in the lower pelvis with their tip projected over the position of the urinary bladder. There is often a radiopaque line along the length of the catheter, so it can be visualised on an X-ray. The inflated urinary catheter balloon is not visualised as it contains water, which is the same density as the urine.

Example

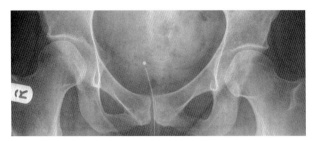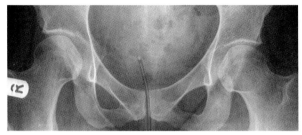

Figure 114: Two identical abdominal radiographs showing a urinary catheter in situ. There is a tube projected over the lower pelvis with its tip projected over the position of the urinary bladder. The right radiograph shows the urinary catheter marked in purple.

Supra-pubic catheter

A supra-pubic catheter is a hollow flexible tube inserted into the urinary bladder via an incision in the **anterior abdominal wall**. The radiographic appearance is similar to that of a normal urinary catheter; however, the catheter is seen to enter the bladder from **above** rather than below.

Example

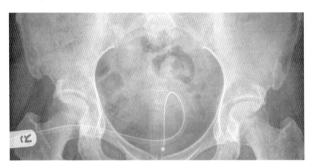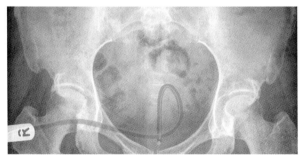

Figure 115: Two identical abdominal radiographs showing a supra-pubic catheter in situ. There is a tube projected over the lower pelvis with its tip pointing inferiorly and projected over the position of the urinary bladder. The right radiograph shows the supra-pubic catheter marked in purple.

E

Nasogastric (NG) and nasojejunal (NJ) tubes

A **nasogastric tube (NG tube)** is a plastic tube inserted through the nose, down the oesophagus and into the stomach. It can be used for short-term feeding, drug administration and aspiration of stomach contents (e.g. for decompression of intestinal obstruction).

Example

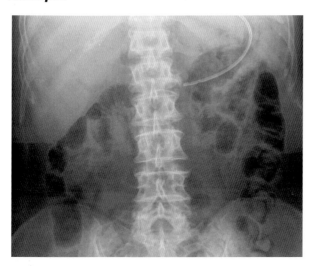 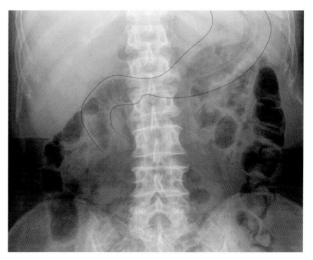

Figure 116: Two identical abdominal radiographs showing a nasogastric (NG) tube in situ. There is a tube projected over the upper abdomen in the region of the stomach. The right radiograph shows the NG tube marked in purple and the approximate position of the stomach marked in brown.

A **nasojejunal tube (NJ tube)** is a plastic tube similar to an NG tube except that it passes through the stomach and duodenum into the jejunum. It is used in individuals unable to tolerate feeding into the stomach.

Example

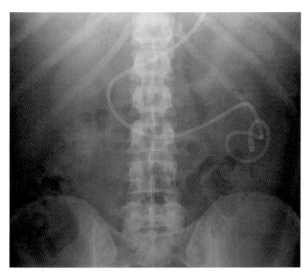 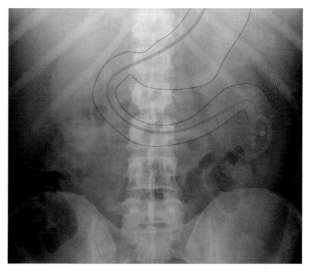

Figure 117: Two identical abdominal radiographs showing a nasojejunal (NJ) tube in situ. There is a tube projected over the upper and mid abdomen, following the curve of the duodenum with its tip to the left of the midline in the region of the proximal jejunum. The right radiograph shows the NJ tube marked in purple and the approximate position of the stomach marked in brown.

E

Flatus tube

A flatus tube is a long soft tube usually inserted into the **sigmoid colon** with the help of a rigid or flexible sigmoidoscope. It is used to decompress a sigmoid volvulus.

Example

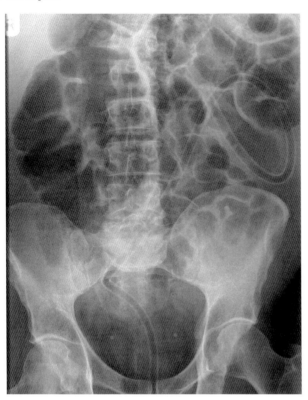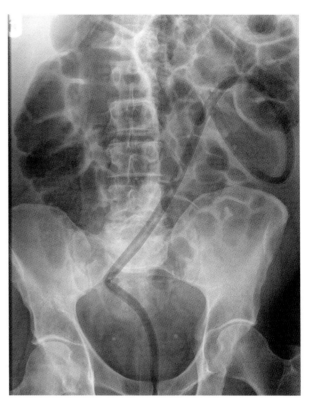

Figure 118: Two identical radiographs showing a flatus tube in situ. There is a large tube projected over the pelvis and lower abdomen, following the path of the rectum and sigmoid colon. The right radiograph shows the flatus tube marked in purple. (You can also see dilated loops of large bowel.)

Surgical drain

Surgical drains come in various shapes and sizes. They are usually used to drain or prevent the accumulation of fluid/blood/pus from the area of surgery.

Example

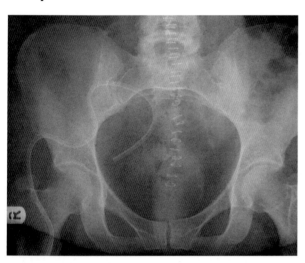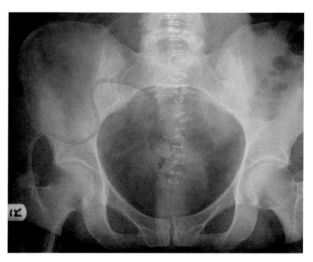

Figure 119: Two identical radiographs showing a simple surgical drain in the pelvis. There is a tube projected over the right pelvis in keeping with a pelvic drain. The right radiograph shows the surgical drain marked in purple. (You can also see midline surgical staples from recent surgery.)

Nephrostomy catheter

A nephrostomy catheter is an artificial connection between the **skin** and **renal pelvis**, usually maintained by a drain, to allow direct **drainage of urine** from the kidney.

Example

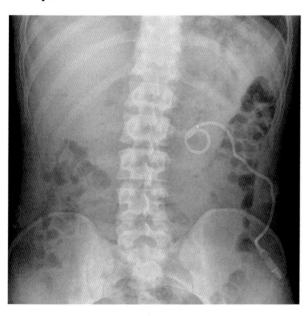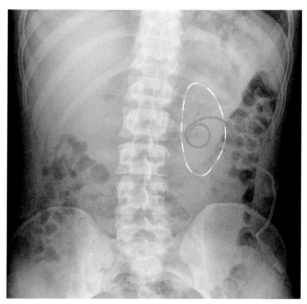

Figure 120: Two identical abdominal radiographs showing a left-sided nephrostomy catheter in situ. There is a left-sided 'pigtail' nephrostomy catheter with a coiled tip (like a pig's tail) projected over the region of the left kidney. The right radiograph shows the left sided nephrostomy catheter marked in purple and the approximate position of the left kidney (not seen clearly) marked with a white dashed line.

Peritoneal dialysis (PD) catheter

A peritoneal dialysis (PD) catheter is placed in the peritoneal cavity and used to **introduce and remove dialysate fluid** for patients undergoing peritoneal dialysis. It is easily recognisable by its large **coiled tip**.

Example

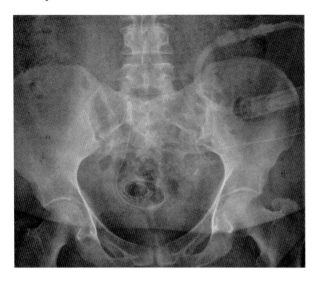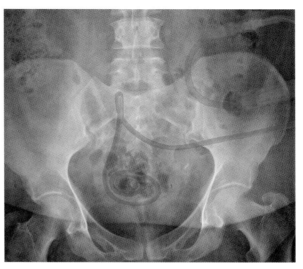

Figure 121: Two identical abdominal radiographs showing a peritoneal dialysis catheter. The coiled tip is seen projected over the pelvis. The right radiograph shows the peritoneal dialysis catheter marked in purple.

Gastric band device

A gastric band device is an **inflatable ring** inserted **surgically** around the top portion of the stomach. It is used as a treatment for obesity by creating a smaller stomach pouch to limit the amount of food that can be consumed at one sitting. The inflatable ring is attached to a small access port placed just under the skin to allow re-adjustment of the band size over time.

Example

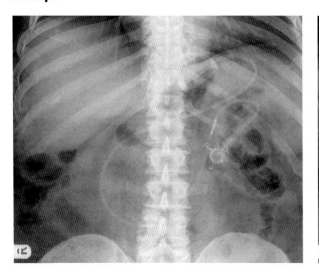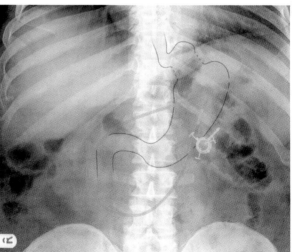

Figure 122: Two identical abdominal radiographs showing a gastric band device in situ. The inflatable ring is projected over the epigastric region (in the correct orientation) and tubing is seen connecting the inflatable ring to the access port. The inflatable ring and tubing are marked in orange and the access port is marked in pink. The approximate position of the stomach is marked in brown.

E

Percutaneous endoscopic gastrostomy (PEG)/radiologically inserted gastrostomy (RIG)

A gastrostomy is a tube passed into the patient's stomach through the abdominal wall. It is used to provide feeding when oral intake is not adequate or safe. A PEG is inserted under endoscopic guidance and a RIG is inserted with radiological (fluoroscopic) guidance.

Example

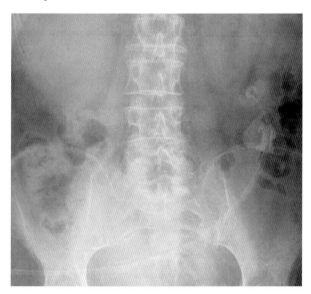 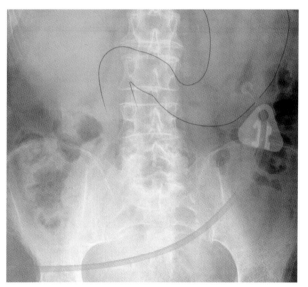

Figure 123: Two identical abdominal radiographs showing a gastrostomy tube in situ. The tubing seen across the lower part of the radiograph is outside the patient, the triangular fixation device is on the skin at the point of entry and the circular tip is within the stomach. The right radiograph shows the gastrostomy marked in orange, the triangular skin fixation device marked in pink and the approximate position of the stomach marked in brown.

Stoma bag

A stoma is a surgically created opening in the abdomen to connect bowel with the outside environment. The three main types are **ileostomy** (small bowel), **colostomy** (large bowel) and **urostomy** (urine via a detached section of ileum). The faeces or urine are collected in a stoma bag attached to the outside of the body over the stoma. On a radiograph you may a see a **dense ring**, which is the site of attachment of the stoma bag to the skin around the stoma.

Example

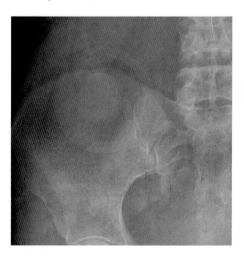 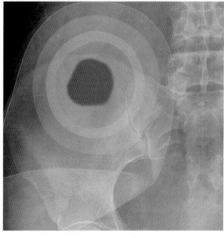

Figure 124: Two identical radiographs of the right lower quadrant showing a stoma bag. There is a dense ring projected over the right lower quadrant in keeping with the skin attachment of the stoma bag. The stoma itself is seen as a dense opacity within the ring of the stoma bag. The stoma bag is marked in pink and the stoma itself is marked in red.

Stents

A stent is a **tube** inserted into a **natural passage** in the body to improve flow or prevent blockage. Below are a few examples of common stents in use:

- **Biliary stent**

Examples

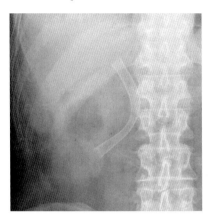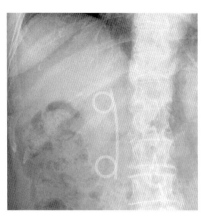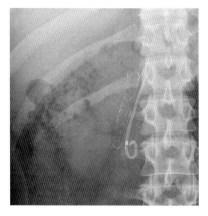

Figure 125: Three different radiographs of the right upper quadrant showing examples of biliary stents. They are placed within the common bile duct and/or hepatic ducts and are usually projected just to the right of the midline in the upper abdomen. The left radiograph shows a metal stent, the middle shows a plastic stent and the right both a metal and plastic stent in situ.

- **Ureteric JJ stent**

Example

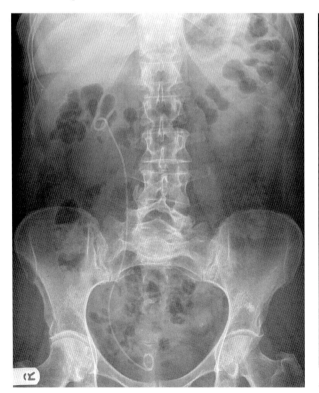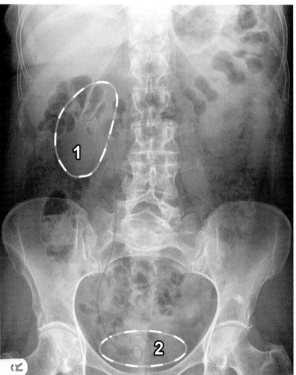

Figure 126: Two identical abdominal radiographs showing a JJ stent in the right ureter. The proximal end is coiled in a loop in the renal pelvis and the distal end is coiled in a loop in the urinary bladder. The 'JJ' in JJ stent refers to the fact that there is a small coil at each end. The right radiograph shows the JJ stent marked in purple, the outline of the right kidney (1) marked with a white dashed line and the approximate outline of the urinary bladder (2) also marked with a white dashed line.

- **Duodenal stent**

  Example

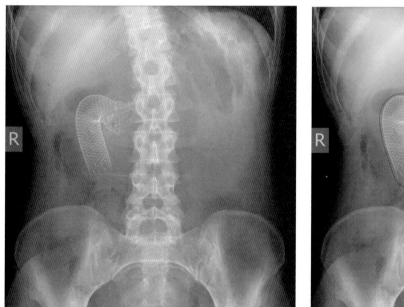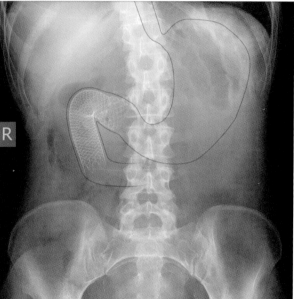

Figure 127: Two identical abdominal radiographs showing a duodenal stent in situ. There is a metallic tubular stent projected over the right side of the abdomen in the position of the duodenum. Given its shape it is likely situated in the first and second parts of the duodenum. It was likely inserted to prevent narrowing from an obstructing tumour. A colonic stent in the hepatic flexure may give a very similar appearance. The right radiograph shows the position of the stomach and duodenum marked in brown.

- **Colonic stent**

  Example

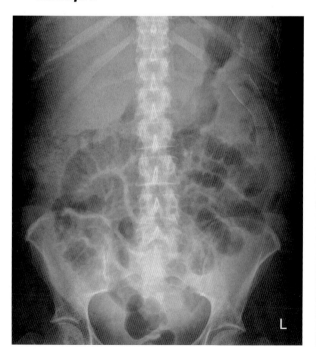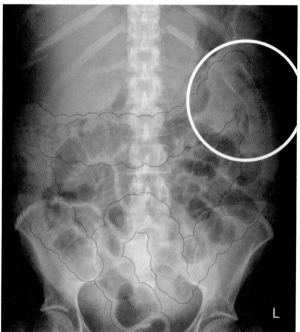

Figure 128: Two identical abdominal radiographs showing a colonic stent in situ. There is a metallic tubular stent projected over the left side of the abdomen in the region of the splenic flexure. It was likely inserted to prevent narrowing from an obstructing tumour. The right radiograph shows the position of the colon marked in brown and the location of the stent marked with a white circle.

- **Endovascular aneurysm repair stent graft**
  An endovascular aneurysm repair (EVAR) is a type of **endovascular surgery** used to treat **AAAs**. A stent graft is placed in the lumen of the aorta to allow blood to flow through and reduce pressure in the aneurysm, preventing rupture (which is associated with a high mortality rate).

Example 1

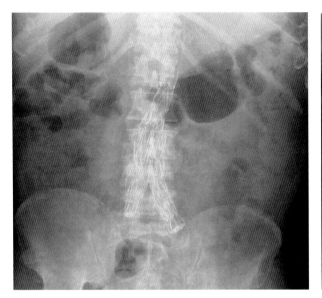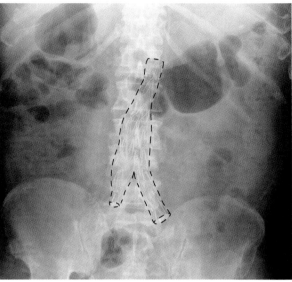

Figure 129: Two identical abdominal radiographs showing an endovascular aneurysm repair (EVAR) stent graft in situ in the abdominal aorta. In this case the endograft is bifurcated extending from the aorta into the left and right common iliac arteries. The right radiograph shows the EVAR stent graft marked in light red.

Example 2

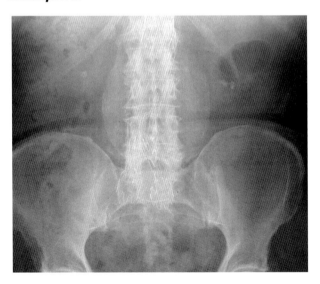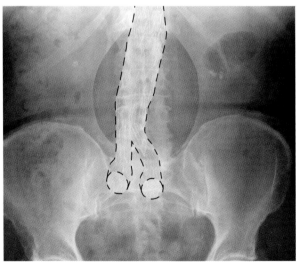

Figure 130: Two identical abdominal radiographs showing an endovascular aneurysm repair (EVAR) stent graft in situ in the abdominal aorta. In this case the endograft is bifurcated extending from the aorta into the left and right common iliac arteries. You can also see the outside edge of the partially calcified abdominal aortic aneurysm (AAA). The right radiograph shows the EVAR stent graft marked in light red and the AAA marked in red.

E

Inferior vena cava (IVC) filter

An inferior vena cava (IVC) filter is an **umbrella-like wire device** placed in the IVC to reduce the risk of large and potentially life threatening **pulmonary emboli**. The wires allow blood to flow past (and small clots), however large clots are prevented from reaching the pulmonary arteries. An IVC filter is often used in situations where anti-coagulation is contraindicated.

Example 1

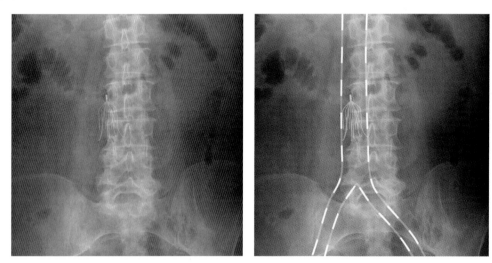

Figure 131: Two identical abdominal radiographs showing an inferior vena cava (IVC) filter in situ. There is an umbrella-like wire device projected just to the right of the midline in the line of the IVC. The right radiograph shows the position of the IVC (not normally visualised) marked in blue with a white outline.

Example 2

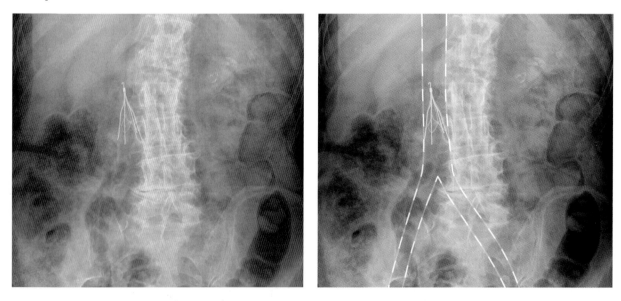

Figure 132: Two identical abdominal radiographs showing another example of an inferior vena cava (IVC) filter in situ. There is an umbrella-like wire device projected just to the right of the midline in the line of the IVC. The right radiograph shows the position of the IVC (not normally visualised) marked in blue with a white outline.

E

Intra-uterine device (IUD)

An intra-uterine device (IUD) is a small device, often '**T'-shaped**, which is inserted into the uterus. They usually contain either copper or levonorgestrel and are commonly used as a form of **long-acting reversible contraception**.

Examples

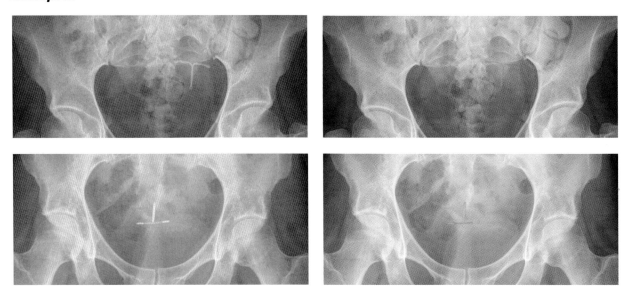

Figure 133: Two sets of two identical abdominal radiographs showing an intra-uterine device (IUD) projected over the pelvic region. The 'T'-shape is typical. The right radiographs show the IUD marked in red.

Pessary

A pessary is a medical device inserted into the **vagina** to provide structural support or to deliver medication. They come in all shapes and sizes, but the most common is the **ring pessary**, which appears as a circular ring projected over the pelvis.

Example

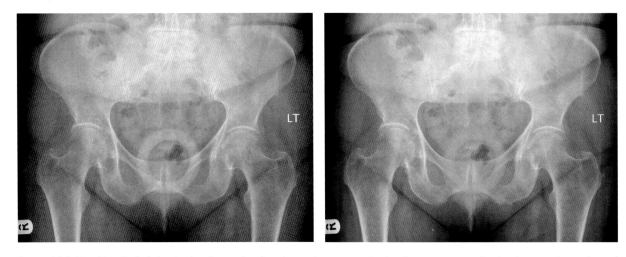

Figure 134: Two identical abdominal radiographs showing a ring pessary in situ. It appears as a circular ring opacity projected over the pelvis. The right radiograph shows the pessary marked in orange.

Foreign bodies

The range and number of different items that can be found on an abdominal radiograph is almost limitless. Key points to keep in mind:

- Artefacts projected over the abdomen may actually be outside of the body (e.g. metal on clothing or items in the patient's pocket)
- Batteries are an important pick up as they are corrosive and can damage the mucosa of the bowel wall. Thankfully they are dense and easily visible.
- Magnets are dangerous as if more than one magnet is swallowed at the same time or a magnet is co-ingested with another metallic object, the loops of intestine can be squeezed between them resulting in bowel perforation.
- Glass is usually visible on plain radiographs.
- Patients insert a variety of foreign bodies into their body orifices with variably plausible explanations. Don't be surprised by some of the things people do.

Retained surgical swab

Example

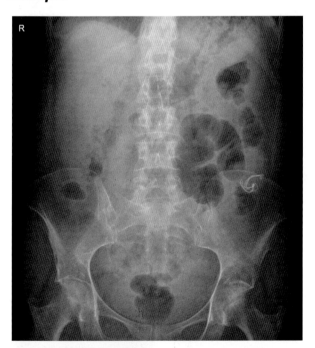
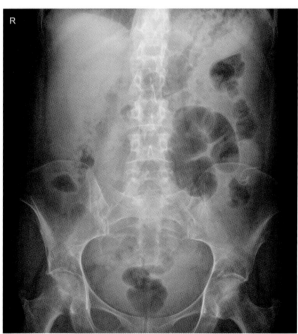

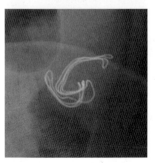
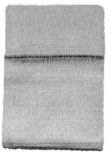

Figure 135: Two identical abdominal radiographs showing a retained surgical swab projected over the left iliac fossa. The radiograph on the right shows the surgical swab marked in red. Surgical swabs usually have an X-ray detectible strand running through them to enable them to be visualised on radiographs. The smaller radiograph to the bottom left shows the X-ray detectible strand more clearly. The image to the bottom right is of a folded surgical swab. You can see the black X-ray detectible strand running through it.

Swallowed objects

Examples

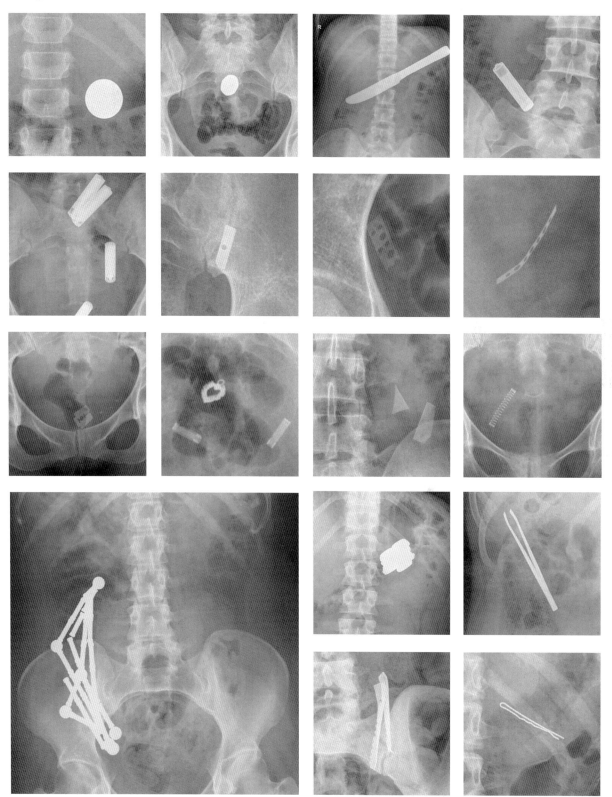

Figure 136: Seventeen radiographs showing swallowed objects. Top row from the left: £1 coin, 50p coin, knife, battery. Second row from the left: batteries, blade, razor blade, razor blade (note the differing appearances). Third row from the left: razor blade, heart shaped locket (and sterilisation clips), shards of glass (note that glass is often visible on plain radiographs), spring from a pen. The large bottom left radiograph shows parts from a magnetic construction toy comprising of rods and balls. Fourth row from the left: cluster of magnets, tweezers. Fifth row from the left: broken alligator type hairclip, hair grip.

E

Examples (continued):

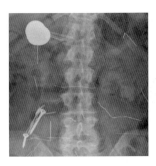 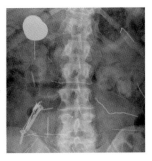 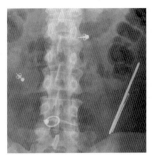 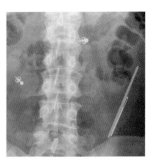

Figure 137: Two sets of two identical radiographs showing various ingested foreign objects. In each case the right hand radiograph shows the objects marked in colour. In the left example there are multiple coins (orange), screws (pink), a hairclip (purple) and many needles and wires. In the right example there are two earrings (yellow), a ring (pink), a rod (red) and a needle (blue).

Objects inserted per-rectum (PR)

Example 1

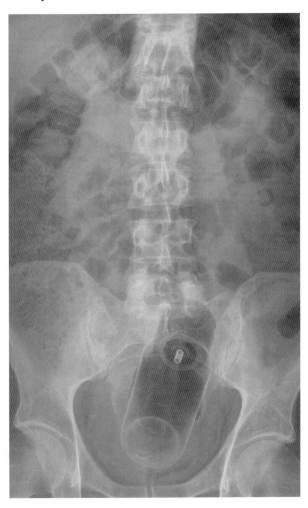 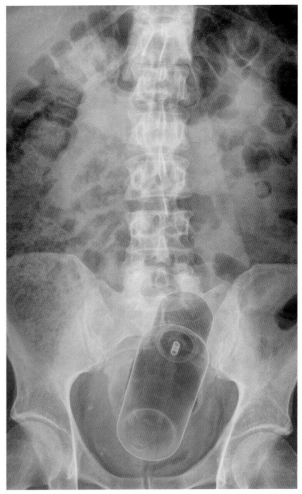

Figure 138: Two identical abdominal radiographs showing a bottle of aftershave which has been inserted into the rectum. The right radiograph shows the bottle marked in green.

Examples 2 and 3

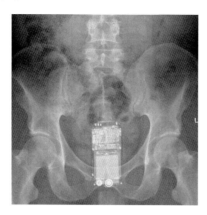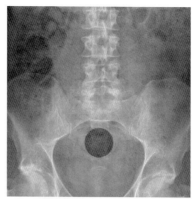

Figure 139: Two different radiographs. The radiograph on the left shows a mobile phone projected over the lower pelvis. This had been inserted into the patient's rectum and needed medical help to remove. The radiograph on the right shows a circular radiolucent foreign body projected over the pelvis in keeping with a ping pong ball.

Example 4

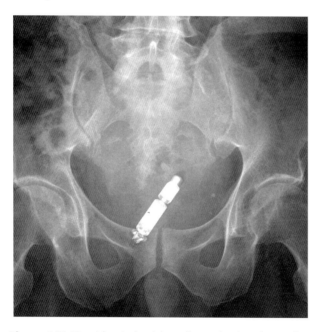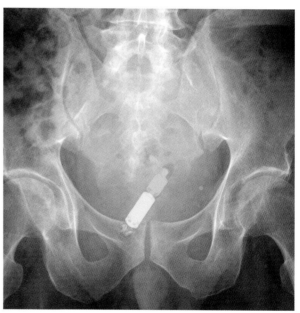

Figure 140: Two identical pelvic radiographs showing a vibrator which has become stuck in the patient's rectum. The right radiograph shows the vibrator marked in purple and battery marked in orange.

E

Clothing artefact

Examples

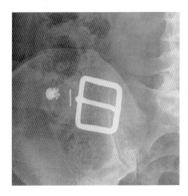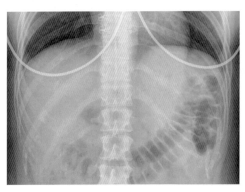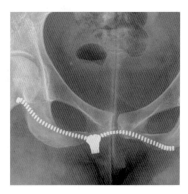

Figure 141: Three radiographs showing different examples of clothing artefact. From left to right they are belt buckle, bra and trouser zip. Ideally these should have been removed prior to taking the X-ray.

Piercings

Examples of umbilical (also called navel or belly button) piercings

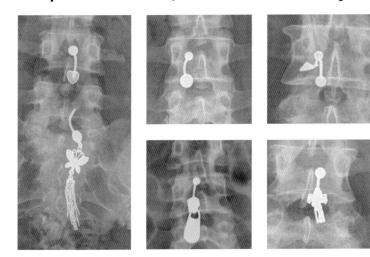

Figure 142: Seven radiographs showing different examples of umbilical (also called navel or belly button) piercings.

Example of clitoral and penile piercings

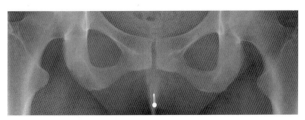

Figure 143: A radiograph of the lower female pelvis showing a clitoral piercing.

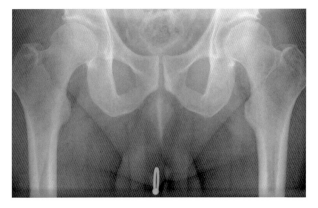

Figure 144: A radiograph of the lower male pelvis showing a penile piercing.

… and finally an example of a tongue piercing that was accidentally swallowed:

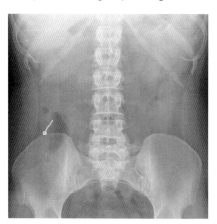 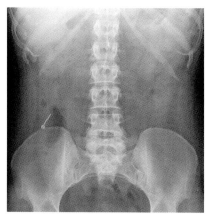

Figure 145: Two identical radiographs showing a tongue piercing that has been accidentally swallowed. The piercing is projected over the right lower quadrant and is likely situated in the large bowel. The right radiograph shows the tongue piercing marked in pink.

Body packer

Body packers smuggle **illicit drugs** by concealing the drugs in their **gastrointestinal tract**. They are sometimes referred to as 'swallowers', 'internal carriers' or 'mules'. The drug is usually densely packed into a balloon, latex glove or condom and swallowed, although insertion of packets into the rectum and vagina has also been reported.

The number of packets may vary from a few to more than 200. Often each packet contains a **potentially life threatening** dose of the drug.

Radiologically the drug packets appear as **multiple oval or tubular soft tissue opacities**, sometimes surrounded by a **rim of gas halo**.

> **Note:** In the past most patients were managed primarily by surgical retrieval however this was associated with significant mortality due to rupture of poorly constructed packages. Most patients nowadays are managed conservatively by using a form of whole bowel irrigation.

E

Example

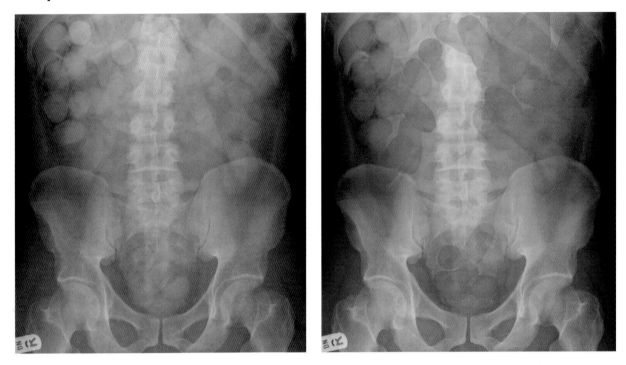

Figure 146: Two identical abdominal radiographs showing multiple oval and tubular shaped soft tissue packets projected over the abdomen. A few have a rim of gas halo surrounding them. These were later found to be condoms containing illicit drugs. The right radiograph shows some of the soft tissue packets marked in purple.

Lung bases

Finally it is important to look at the lung bases (if visualised). In particular look for:

- **Metastasis:** Rounded opacities seen projected over the lung bases.
- **Consolidation:** Patchy opacification at the lung base. A pneumonia (consolidation) at the right lung base may explain a patient's right upper quadrant abdominal pain.
- **Large pleural effusion or lung collapse:** Whiteout at one of the lung bases.

Example 1

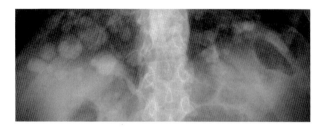 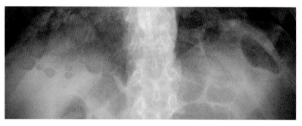

Figure 147: Two identical radiographs of the upper abdomen showing lung metastasis. There are multiple rounded opacities projected over both lung bases most likely in keeping with metastasis. The right radiograph shows the lung metastasis marked in red.

Example 2

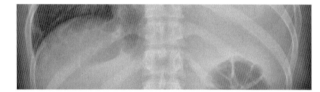 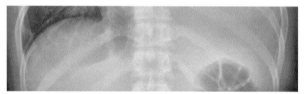

Figure 148: Two identical radiographs of the upper abdomen showing whiteout of the left lung base. There is loss of visualisation of gas (dark) at the left lung base when compared to the right lung base. Possible causes include a large left sided pleural effusion or left lung collapse. The right radiograph shows the whiteout of the left lung base marked in green.

E

Self-assessment questions

These questions test your ability to present an abdominal X-ray and recognise pathology. They are presented in the same format as an objective structured clinical examination (OSCE) or Viva station, so in order to make it as real as possible there are no multiple choice questions (MCQs).

There are 16 questions, each based on one abdominal X-ray. Remember to use the ABCDE approach when presenting and remember there may be **more than one pathology** on a single radiograph.

Part (a) of each question tests your ability to correctly present the X-ray using the ABCDE method and at the same time recognise pathology.

Parts (b) and (c) are typical questions you may get asked in an OSCE and do not necessarily test facts learnt from this book. They are designed to test/teach you more general knowledge relating to the patient's pathology.

The answers can be found on pages 99–106.

Note: Any initials, ages and dates used are purely fictitious and are not related to the patient's X-ray in question.

Example question

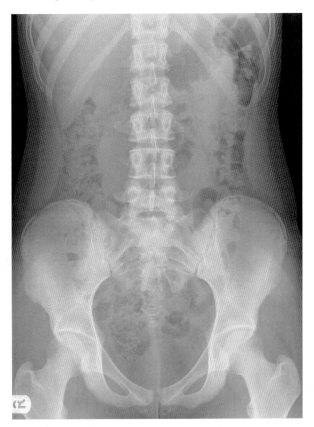

a) Present this radiograph.

"This is a supine AP abdominal radiograph of Mrs VB. The radiograph is anonymised and therefore the date of the examination is unknown."

"The pubic symphysis is included on this radiograph, however the hemi-diaphragms are not visualised. Ideally I would like to see both hemi-diaphragms"

A: "There is no evidence of free gas."

B: "The bowel gas pattern is within normal limits."

C: "There is no abnormal calcification."

D: "There is no fracture or bony abnormality."

E: "There is no evidence of previous surgery, medical devices or any foreign body."

"In summary, this is a normal abdominal radiograph."

Figure 149: Mrs VB. Taken on unknown date.

Abdominal X-rays for Medical Students, First Edition. Christopher G.D. Clarke and Anthony E.W. Dux.

Question 1:

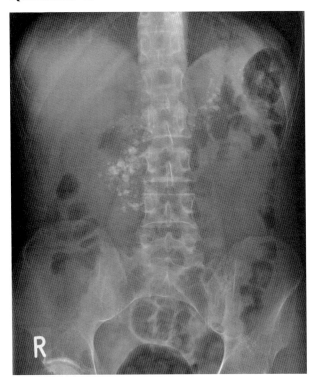

Figure 150: Mr CF. Taken on unknown date.

a) Present this radiograph.
b) What is the diagnosis?
c) Give the most likely underlying cause.

Question 2:

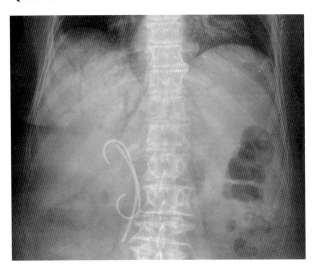

Figure 151: Mr WC. Taken on unknown date.

a) Present this radiograph.
b) Give two indications for the procedure the patient has undergone.
c) Give two specific complications.

Question 3:

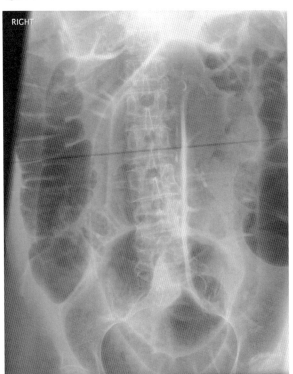

Figure 152: Mrs JV. Taken on unknown date.

a) Present this radiograph.
b) Which age group does this condition commonly affect?
c) What is the initial management?

Question 4:

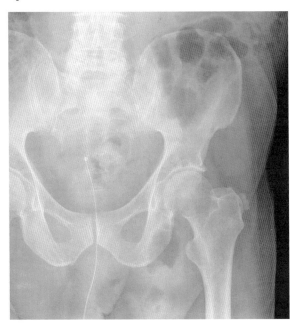

Figure 153: Mr JS. Taken on unknown date.

a) Present this radiograph.
b) What is the most likely diagnosis?
c) Give a complication.

Question 5:

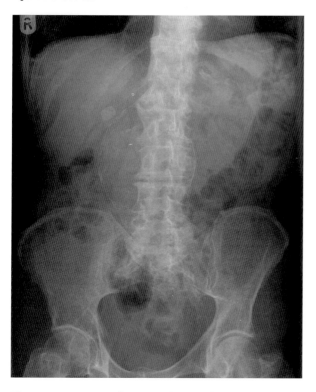

Figure 154: Mr RS. Taken on unknown date.

a) Present this radiograph.
b) What size does an abdominal aortic aneurysm have to be for the risk of spontaneous aneurysm rupture to be larger than the risk of operative management by open surgery or endovascular aneurysm repair (EVAR)?

Question 6:

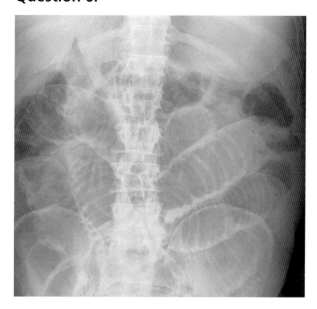

Figure 155: Mr NC. Taken on unknown date.

a) Present this radiograph.
b) What is the diagnosis?
c) What is your initial management plan?

Question 7:

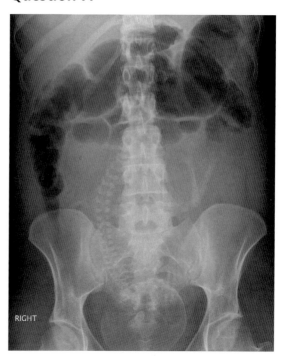

Figure 156: Mrs VN. Taken on unknown date. Severe abdominal pain for 8 h.

a) Present this radiograph.
b) What should have been done prior to this X-ray?
c) The patient was unaware of the pregnancy. What is the next most appropriate investigation?

Question 8:

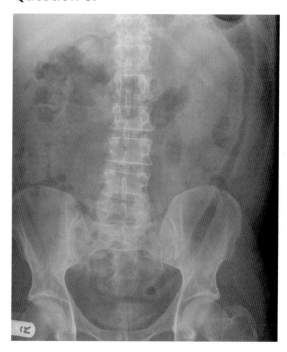

Figure 157: Mrs MB. Taken on unknown date.

a) Present this radiograph.
b) Give three causes for the abnormality shown.
c) List two possible complications.

Question 9:

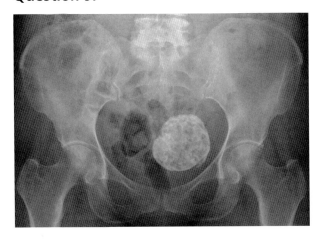

Figure 158: Mrs MH. Taken on unknown date.

a) Present this radiograph.
b) What is demonstrated?
c) In which ethnic group is it more common?

Question 10:

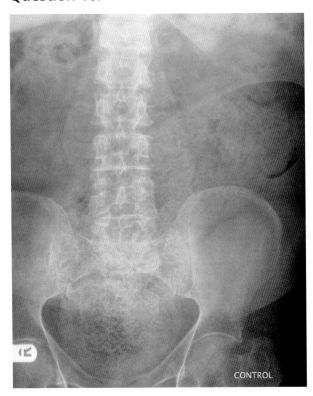

Figure 159: Mrs KH. Taken on unknown date.

a) Present this radiograph.
b) Why might the patient present with diarrhoea?
c) Give two possible complications.

Question 11:

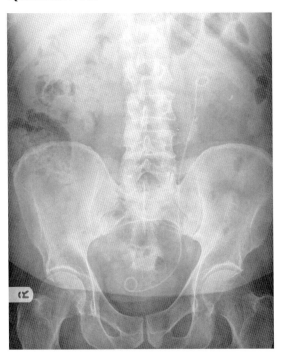

Figure 160: Mr RR. Taken on unknown date.

a) Present this radiograph.
b) Give two indications for the stent shown.

Question 12:

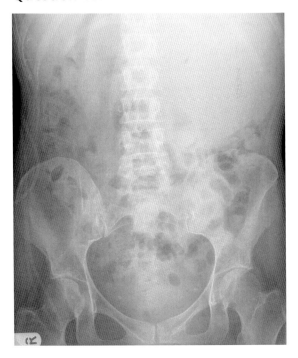

Figure 161: Mrs AT. Taken on unknown date.

a) Present this radiograph.
b) Give two likely underlying causes for this appearance.
c) What investigation would you like to do next?

Question 13:

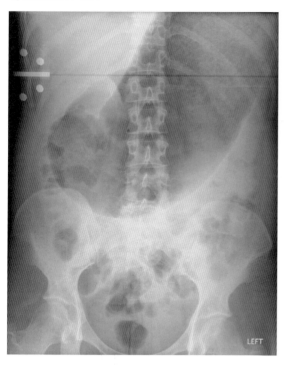

Figure 162: Mrs NM. Taken on unknown date.

a) Present this radiograph.
b) Give two possible causes for this appearance.
c) If the appearances are secondary to bowel obstruction, at what level is the obstruction likely to be?

Question 14:

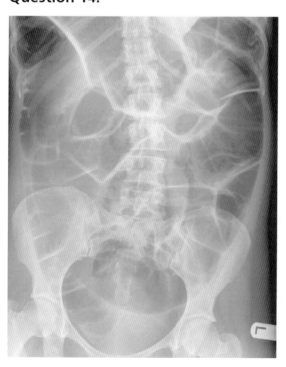

Figure 163: Mrs MS. Taken on unknown date.

a) Present this radiograph.
b) Give two possible causes for this appearance.

Question 15:

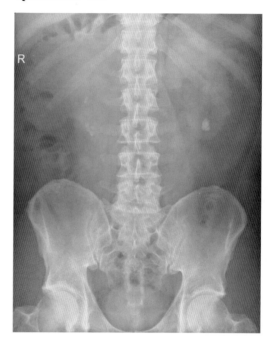

Figure 164: Mr ST. Taken on unknown date.

a) Present this radiograph.
b) What conditions may predispose to these findings?
c) Give one method of treatment.

Question 16

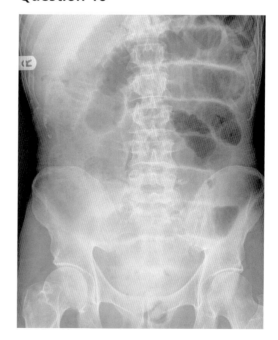

Figure 165: Mrs EA. Taken on unknown date. Abdominal pain and vomiting for 24 h.

a) Present this radiograph.
b) The patient has had previous abdominal surgery. What is the likely cause of the abnormality identified?
c) What is the initial management?

Self-assessment answers

Answer 1:

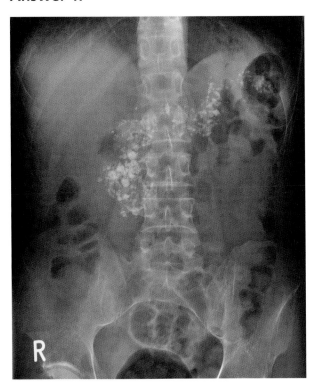

Figure 166: Mr CF. Taken on unknown date (annotated).

a) "This is a supine AP abdominal radiograph of Mr CF. The radiograph is anonymised and therefore the date of the examination is unknown."
   "The hemi-diaphragms are included on this radiograph, however the pubic symphysis is not visualised. Ideally I would like to see the pubic symphysis."
   A: "There is no evidence of free gas."
   B: "The bowel gas pattern is within normal limits."
   C: "There are multiple irregular foci of calcification (marked in yellow) projected over the midline in the mid-abdomen in the rough shape of the pancreas."
   D: "There is no fracture or bony abnormality."
   E: "There is no evidence of previous surgery, medical devices or any foreign body."
   "In summary, this is an abnormal abdominal radiograph showing pancreatic calcification."
b) Chronic calcific pancreatitis.
c) The most likely underlying cause for chronic pancreatitis is alcohol abuse.

Answer 2:

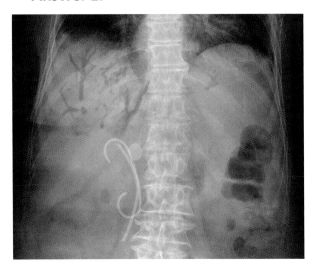

Figure 167: Mr WC. Taken on unknown date (annotated).

a) "This is a supine AP abdominal radiograph of Mr WC. The radiograph is anonymised and therefore the date of the examination is unknown."
   "The hemi-diaphragms are included on this radiograph, however the pubic symphysis is not visualised. Ideally I would like to see the pubic symphysis."
   A: "There are branching dark lines projected over the liver (marked in dark blue), larger and more prominent towards the hilum of the liver."
   B: "The bowel gas pattern is within normal limits."
   C: "There is a rounded calcific density projected over the right upper quadrant (marked in yellow). Given the location this is likely to represent a calcified gallstone."
   D: "There is a wedge fracture of L3."
   E: "There are two short stents projected to the right of the midline in keeping with biliary stents."
   "In summary, this is an abnormal abdominal radiograph showing gas within the biliary tree (pneumobilia), a calcified gallstone, two biliary stents in situ and a wedge fracture of L3."
b) Indications include the following:
   • Palliation or prevention of obstruction from gallstones within the bile duct.
   • Palliation or relief of bile duct obstruction due to pancreatic malignancy.
c) Recognised complications include the following:
   • Perforation of the common bile duct or duodenum.
   • Ascending cholangitis (infection).
   • Pancreatitis.

Abdominal X-rays for Medical Students, First Edition. Christopher G.D. Clarke and Anthony E.W. Dux.
© 2015 John Wiley & Sons, Ltd. Published 2015 by John Wiley & Sons, Ltd.

Answer 3:

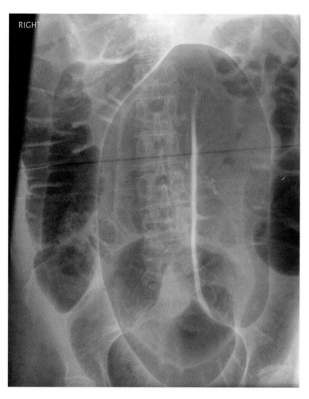

Figure 168: Mrs JV. Taken on unknown date (annotated).

a) "This is a supine AP abdominal radiograph of Mrs JV. The radiograph is anonymised and therefore the date of the examination is unknown."

"The pubic symphysis and hemi-diaphragms are not visualised. Ideally I would like to see both hemi-dia-phragms and pubic symphysis."

A: "There is no evidence of free gas."

B: "There is a 'coffee bean' shaped loop of distended bowel crossing the midline and extending to the right upper quadrant (marked in brown). There is a general lack of haustra within this loop. Further distended loops of bowel are noted in a peripheral location with haustra seen within."

C: "There is no abnormal calcification."

D: "There is no fracture or bony abnormality."

E: "There is no evidence of previous surgery, medical devices or any foreign body."

"In summary, this is an abnormal abdominal radiograph showing a sigmoid volvulus with distension of the ascending, transverse and descending colon."

b) Elderly. There is almost always a history of chronic constipation.

c) Assess the patient's cardiovascular status and give intravenous (IV) fluids. Insert a flatus tube per rectum to decompress the dilated bowel.

Answer 4:

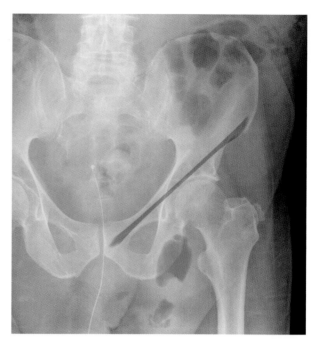

Figure 169: Mr JS. Taken on unknown date (annotated).

a) "This is a supine AP pelvic radiograph of Mr JS. The radiograph is anonymised and therefore the date of the examination is unknown."

"The pubic symphysis is included on this radiograph, however the hemi-diaphragms and upper abdomen are not visualised. Ideally I would like to see both hemi-diaphragms."

A: "There is no evidence of free gas."

B: "There is a loop of gas filled bowel (marked in green) projected over the left groin area below and lateral to the left obturator foramen and below the level of the inguinal ligament (marked in grey)."

C: "There is no abnormal calcification."

D: "There is no fracture or bony abnormality."

E: "There is a urinary catheter in situ."

"In summary, this is an abnormal abdominal radiograph showing a left groin hernia and urinary catheter in situ."

b) Large left inguinal hernia. Inguinal hernias are more common than femoral hernias in male patients.

c) Possible correct answers include the following:

• Obstruction – If the herniated loop of bowel becomes trapped or tightly pinched at the point where it protrudes through the abdominal wall, the loop of bowel may become obstructed.

• Strangulation – Rarely, the hernia traps the bowel so tightly that the blood supply to the bowel is compromised. This is a serious complication and may lead to gangrene, bowel rupture, peritonitis and, if untreated, death.

Answer 5:

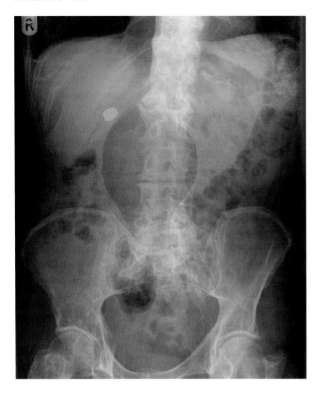

Figure 170: Mr RS. Taken on unknown date (annotated).

a) "This is a supine AP abdominal radiograph of Mr RS. The radiograph is anonymised and therefore the date of the examination is unknown."

"The hemi-diaphragms are included on this radiograph, however the pubic symphysis is only partially visualised. Ideally I would like to see the pubic symphysis."

A: "There is no evidence of free gas."

B: "The bowel gas pattern is within normal limits."

C: "There is a large dilated vascular structure in the midline with wall calcification seen (marked in red). It measures over 3 cm in diameter. There is also a well defined calcified opacity with a polygonal shape projected over the right upper quadrant in the region of the gallbladder (marked in yellow). A further area of linear calcification is seen projected over the left upper quadrant with a tortuous 'Chinese Dragon' like appearance outlining the splenic artery."

D: "There is degenerative change in the spine."

E: "There is no evidence of previous surgery, medical devices or any foreign body."

"In summary, this is an abnormal abdominal radiograph showing an abdominal aortic aneurysm (AAA), a calcified gallstone projected over the right upper quadrant and degenerative change in the spine. Incidental splenic artery calcification noted."

b) >5.5 cm diameter. At this size the risk of aneurysm rupture outweighs the risk of operative management, and treatment is recommended.

Answer 6:

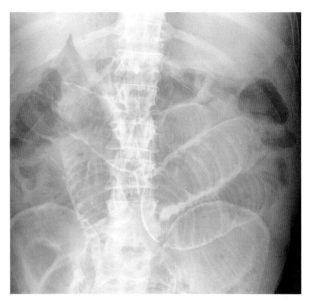

Figure 171: Mr NC. Taken on unknown date (annotated).

a) "This is a supine AP abdominal radiograph of Mr NC. The radiograph is anonymised and therefore the date of the examination is unknown."

"The pubic symphysis and hemi-diaphragms are not visualised. Ideally I would like to see both hemi-diaphragms and pubic symphysis."

A: "There is gas outlining both sides of the bowel wall (lumen of bowel marked in brown and free gas marked in turquoise) in keeping with Rigler's sign."

B: "There are multiple centrally located gas-filled loops of bowel. Valvulae conniventes are seen in many of the loops and they measure >3 cm in diameter in keeping with dilated loops of small bowel."

C: "There is no abnormal calcification."

D: "There is no fracture or bony abnormality."

E: "There is no evidence of previous surgery, medical devices or any foreign body."

"In summary, this is an abnormal abdominal radiograph showing a pneumoperitoneum and dilated loops of small bowel."

b) Bowel perforation.

c) Assess the clinical status of the patient and resuscitate as necessary. Urgently refer the patient to the general surgeons. Give intravenous (IV) fluids, insert an NG tube and make the patient nil by mouth. Give broad-spectrum antibiotics and analgesia. If the patient is stable, consider a computed tomography (CT) scan to look for an underlying cause.

Answer 7:

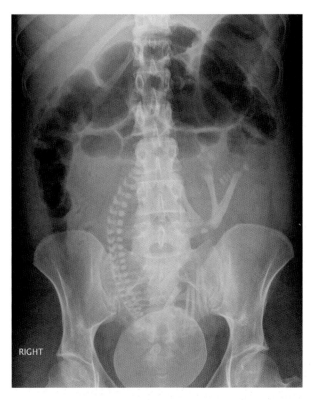

Figure 172: Mrs VN. Taken on unknown date (annotated).

a) "This is a supine AP abdominal radiograph of Mrs VN. The radiograph is anonymised and therefore the date of the examination is unknown."

"The pubic symphysis and hemi-diaphragms are not visualised. Ideally I would like to see both hemi-dia-phragms and pubic symphysis."

A: "There is no evidence of free gas."

B: "The bowel gas pattern is within normal limits."

C: "There is abnormal calcification seen projected over the lower abdomen and pelvis with appearances in keeping with a fetus (marked in yellow). The spine of the fetus is seen to the right of the midline; lower limbs in the centre of the abdomen; upper limbs projected over the sacrum and the fetal skull in the pelvis."

D: "There is no fracture or bony abnormality."

E: "There is no evidence of previous surgery, medical devices or any foreign body."

"In summary, this is an abnormal abdominal radiograph showing a fetus in situ."

b) The radiographer should have asked the patient if there is any chance she should be pregnant, and a pregnancy test should have been performed if the patient was unsure.

c) Ultrasound scan of the abdomen to assess the foetus.

Answer 8:

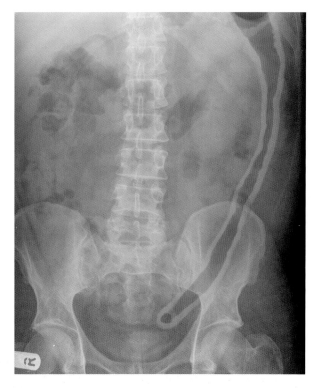

Figure 173: Mrs MB. Taken on unknown date (annotated).

a) "This is a supine AP abdominal radiograph of Mrs MB. The radiograph is anonymised and therefore the date of the examination is unknown."

"The hemi-diaphragms are not visualised and the pubic symphysis is only partially visualised. Ideally I would like to see both the hemi-diaphragms and the pubic symphysis."

A: "There is no evidence of free gas."

B: "The descending colon appears featureless with loss of the normal haustra giving a 'lead pipe' appearance (marked in green). There is also thickening of the bowel wall (marked in light green)."

C: "There is no abnormal calcification."

D: "There is no fracture or bony abnormality."

E: "There is no evidence of previous surgery, medical devices or any foreign body."

"In summary, this is an abnormal abdominal radiograph showing bowel wall inflammation of the descending colon with a 'lead pipe' appearance."

b) • Inflammatory bowel disease
   • Ischaemic bowel
   • Infection

c) Specific complications will vary depending on the underlying cause of the colitis. Possible correct answers include, but are not limited to the following:
   • Intestinal perforation
   • Severe bleeding per rectum
   • Colonic strictures

Answer 9:

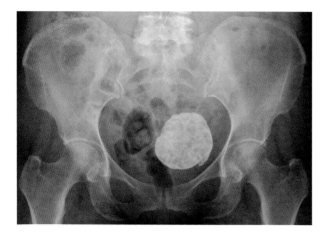

Figure 174: Mrs MH. Taken on unknown date (annotated).

a) "This is a supine AP pelvic radiograph of Mrs MH. The radiograph is anonymised and therefore the date of the examination is unknown."

"The pubic symphysis is included on this radiograph, however the hemi-diaphragms are not visualised. Ideally I would like to see both hemi-diaphragms."

A: "There is no evidence of free gas."

B: "The bowel gas pattern is within normal limits."

C: "There is a large rounded area of calcification projected over the left pelvis with irregular areas of calcification within (marked in yellow). Appearances are typical of a calcified uterine fibroid."

D: "There is no fracture or bony abnormality."

E: "There is no evidence of previous surgery, medical devices or any foreign body."

"In summary, this is an abnormal abdominal radiograph showing a large calcified uterine fibroid."

b) Uterine fibroid (uterine leiomyoma).

c) Afro-Caribbean women (3× more common).

Answer 10:

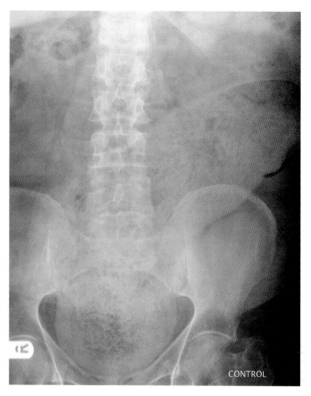

Figure 175: Mrs KH. Taken on unknown date (annotated).

a) "This is a supine AP abdominal radiograph of Mrs KH. The radiograph is anonymised and therefore the date of the examination is unknown."

"The hemi-diaphragms are not visualised and the pubic symphysis is only partially visualised. Ideally I would like to see both the hemi-diaphragms and the pubic symphysis."

A: "There is no evidence of free gas."

B: "There is a huge volume of faecal material extending from the pelvis to the left upper quadrant in keeping with a huge faecal impaction causing massive distension of the rectum (marked in brown)."

C: "There is no abnormal calcification."

D: "There is no fracture or bony abnormality."

E: "There is no evidence of previous surgery, medical devices or any foreign body."

"In summary, this is an abnormal abdominal radiograph showing a large faecal impaction."

b) In some patients the liquid stool passes around the obstruction (impacted faeces) giving paradoxical or overflow diarrhoea.

c) Possible correct answers include the following:
  • Ulceration or necrosis of rectal tissue
  • Bowel incontinence
  • Bleeding from anus

Answer 11:

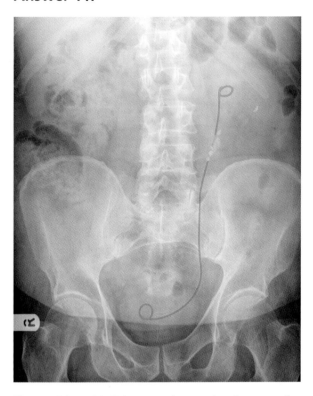

Figure 176: Mr RR. Taken on unknown date (annotated).

a) "This is a supine AP abdominal radiograph of Mr RR. The radiograph is anonymised and therefore the date of the examination is unknown."

"The pubic symphysis is included on this radiograph, however the hemi-diaphragms are not visualised. Ideally I would like to see both hemi-diaphragms."

A: "There is no evidence of free gas."

B: "The bowel gas pattern is within normal limits."

C: "There are multiple small calcific densities projected to the left of the lumbar spine (marked in yellow). These are most likely in keeping with ureteric calculi as they are projected over the line of the left ureter. The term 'steinstrasse' (literally 'stone street') may be used for this appearance, which is often seen post-lithotripsy. A small calcific density is also projected over the lower pole of the left kidney in keeping with a renal calculus (also marked in yellow)."

D: "There is no fracture or bony abnormality."

E: "There is a JJ stent in the left ureter (marked in purple)."

"In summary, this is an abnormal abdominal radiograph showing multiple left sided ureteric calculi, a small calculus at the lower pole of the left kidney and JJ stent in the left ureter."

b) Main indications:

- Relieve obstructive uropathy (e.g. obstructing renal calculus)
- Post surgery to allow healing of the ureter and prevent stricture formation

Answer 12:

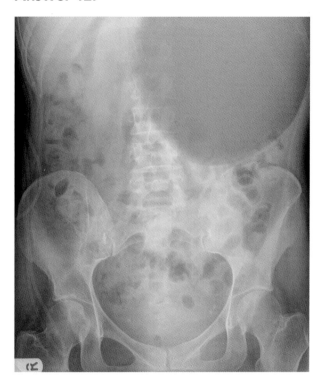

Figure 177: Mrs AT. Taken on unknown date (annotated).

a) "This is a supine AP abdominal radiograph of Mrs AT. The radiograph is anonymised and therefore the date of the examination is unknown."

"The pubic symphysis is included on this radiograph, however the hemi-diaphragms are not visualised. Ideally I would like to see both hemi-diaphragms."

A: "There is no evidence of free gas."

B: "The bowel gas pattern is within normal limits."

C: "There is no abnormal calcification."

D: "There is a large rounded soft tissue density in the left upper quadrant displacing loops of bowel inferiorly and medially (marked in red)."

E: "There is no evidence of previous surgery, medical devices or any foreign body. Some tubing is seen projected at the edge of the radiograph on the right side, likely external to the patient."

"In summary, this is an abnormal abdominal radiograph showing a large soft tissue mass in the left upper quadrant."

b) Splenomegaly or left renal mass are likely given the location.

c) Ultrasound scan of the abdomen. This can be performed relatively quickly and does not involve ionising radiation. If ultrasound cannot diagnose the mass then a CT scan of the abdomen and pelvis with intravenous contrast is the next most appropriate investigation.

Answer 13:

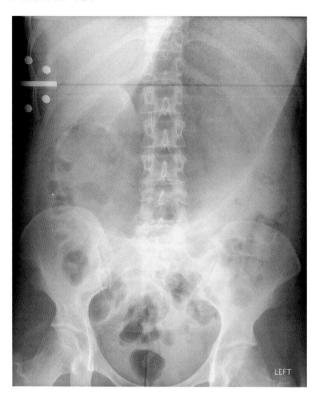

Figure 178: Mrs NM. Taken on unknown date (annotated).

a) "This is a supine AP abdominal radiograph of Mrs NM. The radiograph is anonymised and therefore the date of the examination is unknown."

   "The pubic symphysis and hemi-diaphragms are not visualised. Ideally I would like to see both hemi-diaphragms and pubic symphysis."

   A: "There is no evidence of free gas."

   B: "There is a large loop of stomach shaped distended bowel in the upper abdomen (marked in light blue)."

   C: "There is no abnormal calcification."

   D: "There is no fracture or bony abnormality."

   E: "There is no evidence of previous surgery, medical devices or any foreign body."

   "In summary, this is an abnormal abdominal radiograph showing a gas filled dilated stomach."

b) Bowel obstruction (e.g. due to malignancy or due to scarring in the duodenum from peptic ulcer disease) or aerophagia (e.g. distressed patients or as a side effect of non-invasive ventilation).

c) Stomach pylorus/proximal duodenum as the bowel distal to this point is not distended.

Answer 14:

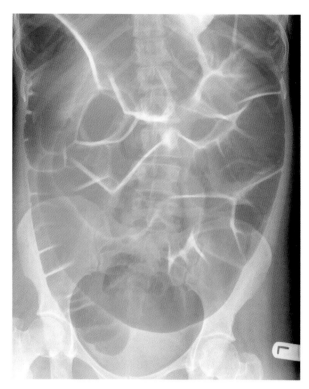

Figure 179: Mrs MS. Taken on unknown date (annotated).

a) "This is a supine AP abdominal radiograph of Mrs MS. The radiograph is anonymised and therefore the date of the examination is unknown."

   "The hemi-diaphragms are not visualised and the pubic symphysis is only partially visualised. Ideally I would like to see both the hemi-diaphragms and the pubic symphysis."

   A: "There is no evidence of free gas."

   B: "There are multiple dilated loops of large bowel measuring over 5.5 cm in diameter with haustra seen within (marked in green)."

   C: "There is no abnormal calcification."

   D: "There is no fracture or bony abnormality."

   E: "There is no evidence of previous surgery, medical devices or any foreign body."

   "In summary, this is an abnormal abdominal radiograph showing multiple dilated loops of large bowel."

b) Correct answers include the following:
   • Malignancy – Colorectal carcinoma is the most common cause of large bowel obstruction in adults.
   • Diverticular structure

   Other causes of large bowel obstruction include a volvulus (there is no evidence of a volvulus in this radiograph) and faecal impaction (there is no evidence of impacted faeces on this radiograph).

Answer 15:

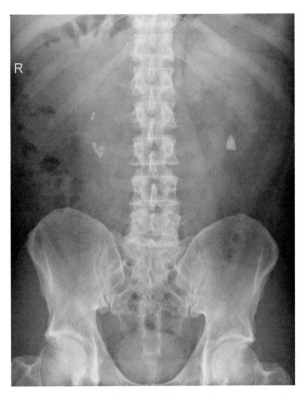

Figure 180: Mr ST. Taken on unknown date (annotated).

a) "This is a supine AP abdominal radiograph of Mr ST. The radiograph is anonymised and therefore the date of the examination is unknown."

"The pubic symphysis and hemi-diaphragms are not visualised. Ideally I would like to see both hemi-dia-phragms and pubic symphysis."

A: "There is no evidence of free gas."

B: "The bowel gas pattern is within normal limits."

C: "There are a few small calcific densities projected to the left and right of the lumbar spine (marked in yellow). The left sided calcific densities are projected over the lower pole of the left kidney and the right sided calcific densities are projected over the mid and lower pole of the right kidney."

D: "There is no fracture or bony abnormality."

E: "There is no evidence of previous surgery, medical devices or any foreign body."

"In summary, this is an abnormal abdominal radiograph showing bilateral renal calculi."

b) Correct answers include (but are not limited to):
- Urinary tract infections (chronic)
- Hyperparathyroidism
- Hypercalciuria
- Cystinuria
- Anatomical anomalies (e.g. horseshoe kidney)

c) Correct answers include (but are not limited to) the following:
- Extracorporeal shock wave lithotripsy (ESWL)
- Percutaneous nephropyelolithotomy

Answer 16:

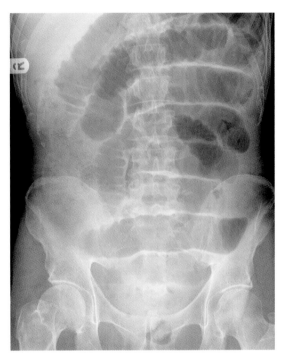

Figure 181: Mrs EA. Taken on unknown date. Abdominal pain and vomiting for 24h (annotated).

a) "This is a supine AP abdominal radiograph of Mrs EA. The radiograph is anonymised and therefore the date of the examination is unknown."

"The pubic symphysis is included on this radiograph, however the hemi-diaphragms are not visualised. Ideally I would like to see both hemi-diaphragms."

A: "There is no evidence of free gas."

B: "There are multiple centrally located gas-filled loops of bowel (marked in blue). Valvulae conniventes are seen in many of the loops and they measure >3cm in diameter in keeping with dilated loops of small bowel."

C: "There is no abnormal calcification."

D: "There is no fracture or bony abnormality."

E: "There is no evidence of previous surgery, medical devices or any foreign body."

"In summary, this is an abnormal abdominal radiograph showing dilated loops of small bowel."

b) Mechanical small bowel obstruction secondary to adhesions (most common in the UK).

c) 'Drip and suck'. Drip=give intravenous (IV) fluids, suck=insert nasogastric (NG) tube and make the patient nil by mouth. Urgently refer the patient to the general surgeons. Consider a CT scan to look for an underlying cause. If the bowel obstruction does not resolve within 24–28h, surgery may be required.

Glossary

Abscess – A localised collection of pus surrounded by inflamed tissue

Adhesion – Fibrous band that forms between tissues and organs, often as a result of injury during surgery

Aerophagia – Excessive air swallowing

Aetiology – The cause or origin of a disease

Anastomosis – The connection of two luminal structures (e.g. two loops of bowel)

Aneurysm – Abnormal localised enlargement (dilation) of an artery

Anterior – Located in front of or towards the front of a structure

Anterior–posterior (AP) – The X-ray tube is placed in front of the patient and the X-rays pass in the AP direction

AXR – Abdominal X-ray

Benign – Not recurrent or progressive; not malignant

Bilateral – Involving both sides

Biliary – Relating to bile or the bile duct

Calcification – The process by which calcium builds up in soft tissues

Calculus – A stone in the kidney or urinary tract (*plural: calculi*)

Carcinogenesis – Transformation of normal cells into cancer cells

Carcinoma – A malignant tumour derived from epithelial tissue

Catheter – A hollow tube inserted into a body cavity, duct or vessel to withdraw or insert fluid

Cholangitis – Inflammation of the bile ducts

Cholecystitis – Inflammation of the gallbladder

Circumferential – Encircling or pertaining to a circumference

Colitis – Inflammation of the colon

Collection – In the context of radiology, usually refers to a localised area of fluid or pus

Colon – The section of the large intestine extending from the caecum to the rectum

Computed tomography – A medical imaging technique that uses X-rays to produce a detailed image of a cross section of tissue

Congenital – Present or existing at the time of birth

Constipation – Difficult, incomplete, or infrequent evacuation of dry, hardened faeces from the bowels

Contrast – The degree to which light and dark areas of an image differ because of the differences in absorption between one tissue and another

Contrast medium/agent – An administered radiopaque substance (e.g. barium or iodine-based compounds) used in radiology to permit visualisation of internal body structures

Cortex (of the kidney) – The outer layer of the kidney

Costal – Pertaining to a rib

Costophrenic angle – The angle between the ribs and the diaphragm on a chest radiograph

Crohn's disease – A type of inflammatory bowel disease that may affect any part of the gastrointestinal tract from mouth to anus

CT – *See* **computed tomography**

Cystinuria – An inherited autosomal recessive disease characterised by the formation of cystine stones in the kidneys, ureter and bladder

Decubitus – *See* **lateral decubitus**

Density – The mass per unit volume

Diaphragm – The musculo-membranous partition separating the thoracic and abdominal cavities and acting as the major muscle for inspiration

Dilatation – The act of dilating or stretching

Abdominal X-rays for Medical Students, First Edition. Christopher G.D. Clarke and Anthony E.W. Dux.
© 2015 John Wiley & Sons, Ltd. Published 2015 by John Wiley & Sons, Ltd.

Distal – Away from or the farthest from a point of origin or attachment

Diverticulitis – Inflammation of the diverticula along the wall of the colon

Diverticulum – An abnormal small, blind-ending pouch opening from a hollow or fluid-filled viscous, for example colon or bladder (*plural:* **diverticula***, adjective:* **diverticular**)

Duodenum – The first portion of the small intestine, from the stomach to the jejunum

Electromagnetic radiation – A form of energy exhibiting wave-like behaviour as it travels through space. It is classified according to the frequency of its wave

Electromagnetic spectrum – The range of all possible frequencies of electromagnetic radiation

Emphysematous – Any abnormal distension of an organ, or part of the body, with air or other gas

Endoscopic retrograde cholangio pancreatography – A test that combines the use of a flexible endoscope with fluoroscopy to examine the biliary tract and perform certain procedures including gallstone removal and biliary stent insertion

Endoscopy – An examination by means of an endoscope, an instrument used to examine the interior of a hollow organ or cavity of the body

Endovascular aneurysm repair – A type of endovascular surgery used to treat abdominal aortic aneurysms (AAAs). A stent graft is placed in the lumen of the aorta to allow blood to flow through and reduce pressure in the aneurysm, preventing rupture

Enteric – Intestinal

Epigastric – Pertaining to the epigastrium, the upper middle part of the abdomen

ERCP – *See* **endoscopic retrograde cholangio pancreatography**

Erect – Upright in position or posture

EVAR – *See* **endovascular aneurysm repair**

Expiration – Breathing out

Exposure – The quantifiable dose of radiation on a subject; the number of X-rays that reach the detector and make the image

Extracorporeal shock wave lithotripsy (ESWL) – A non-invasive treatment of kidney stones (renal calculi) using high energy ultrasound waves

Falciform ligament – A ligament attaching the liver to the anterior abdominal wall (a remnant of the umbilical vein)

Femoral – Of or relating to the thigh or femur

Fibroid – *See* **uterine fibroid**

Fistula – An abnormal passageway between two organs in the body or between an organ and the exterior of the body

Fluoroscopy – An imaging technique that uses X-rays to obtain real-time moving images of the internal structures of a patient

Foci – *See* **focus**

Focus – The primary centre from which a disease develops or in which it localizes (*plural:* **Foci**)

Foetus – An unborn human more than 8 weeks after conception

Foreign body – Any object originating outside the body

Gallstone – A small, hard, pathological concretion of cholesterol, bile pigments, and lime salts, formed in the gallbladder or in a bile duct

Gangrene – Localised death and decomposition of body tissue caused by a lack of blood supply

Gastrointestinal – Of or relating to the stomach or intestines

Gastroparesis – Delayed gastric emptying

Gland – An aggregation of cells specialised to synthesise a substance for release such as hormones

Granular – Resembling or consisting of small grains or particles

Granulomatous – Composed of granulomas, localised masses of inflamed granulation tissue

Haemostatic – An agent used to reduce or stop bleeding from blood vessels

Haustra – Small pouches in the wall of the large intestine. They have a characteristic appearance on an abdominal radiograph (*see page 34*)

Hemi-diaphragm – Half of the diaphragm, the muscle that separates the chest cavity from the abdomen and that serves as the main muscle of inspiration

Hilum – A depression or recess on an organ through which blood vessels, nerves and ducts enter and leave

Homogenous – Uniform in structure or composition throughout

Hypercalciuria – Excess of calcium in the urine

Hyperparathyroidism – The overproduction of parathyroid hormone from the parathyroid glands

Hypochondrium – The upper lateral abdominal region, overlying the costal cartilages on either side of the epigastrium

Iatrogenic – Caused by medical examination or treatment

Ileocecal valve – A physiological valve between the ileum and caecum of the large bowel; it prevents material flowing back from the large to the small intestine

Ileus – Disruption of the normal propulsive ability of the gastrointestinal tract (i.e. failure of peristalsis)

Inferior – Lower in place or position, the opposite of superior

Inflammation – The reaction of living tissues to injury or infection, characterised by heat, redness, swelling and pain

Inguinal – Pertaining to the groin

Inguinal ligament – A fibrous band running from the anterior superior iliac spine of the ilium to the pubic tubercle of the pubic bone

Intussusception – The enfolding of one segment of the intestine within another, often causing pain and bowel obstruction

Ionisation – The process in which a neutral atom or molecule gains or loses electrons and thus acquires a negative or positive electrical charge. Ionising radiation produces ionisation in its passage through body tissue or other matter. Ionisation can cause cell death or mutation (*plural*: **ionisations**)

IRMER 2000 – The Ionising Radiation (Medical Exposure) Regulations 2000. Introduced in 2000, it lays down the basic measures for radiation protection for patients in the UK

Ischaemia – Insufficient supply of blood to an organ or tissues, usually due to a blocked artery

Laparotomy – A surgical procedure involving a large incision through the abdominal wall to gain access to the abdominal cavity

Lateral – Situated at the side, away from the middle, extending away from the median plane of the body

Lateral decubitus – Patient lying on their side (e.g. left lateral decubitus = patient lying on their left side)

Lesion – A general term referring to almost any abnormality involving any tissue or organ

Lucent – *See* **radiolucent**

Lumen – The inner open space or cavity of a tube for example blood vessel or intestine

Lymph nodes – Small glands found throughout the body; they are a part of the lymphatic system and play a major role in the immune system

Malignancy – Cancerous cells that have the ability to spread to other sites in the body (metastasise) or to invade and destroy tissues

Medial – Situated in the middle, extending towards the middle, closer to the middle/median plane of the body

Medulla (of the kidney) – The inner part of the kidney, chiefly comprising collecting tubules and organised into a group of structures called the medullary pyramids

Medullary pyramids – *See* **medulla** (of the kidney)

Medullary sponge kidney – A congenital disorder of the kidneys characterised by cystic dilation of the collecting ducts and in most cases patients develop medullary nephrocalcinosis

Megacolon – *See* **toxic megacolon**

Mesenteric – Pertaining to the mesentery

Mesentery (of the bowel) – The double layer of peritoneum containing blood vessels, lymph vessels and nerves, which suspends parts of the bowel from the posterior wall of the abdomen

Metastasis – The process by which a cancer spreads from the place at which it first arose as a primary tumour to distant locations in the body; the cancer resulting from the spread of the primary tumour

Metastatic – Relating to metastasis

Mitotic – Relating to cell division

Mottled – Spotted or blotched with different shades

Mucosal – Relating to the mucosa or mucous membrane, the lining of the digestive and respiratory tracts

Mutation – A change in the structure of the genes or chromosomes of an organism

Nasogastric (NG) – Referring to the passage from the nose to the stomach

Nasogastric (NG) tube – A tube that is passed through the nose down into the stomach

Nasojejunal (NJ) – Referring to the passage from the nose to the jejunum

Nasojejunal (NJ) tube – A tube that is passed through the nose down into the jejunum

Necrotising enterocolitis (NEC) – An acute inflammatory disease occurring in the intestines of premature infants. Necrosis of intestinal tissue may follow

Nephropyelolithotomy – Laparoscopic removal of calculus from the renal pelvis

Neurogenic – Originating in the nerves or nervous tissue

NG – *See* **nasogastric (NG)**

NJ – *See* **nasojejunal (NJ)**

Obturator foramen – The opening created between the ischium and pubis bones of the pelvis

Oddi – *See* **sphincter of Oddi**

Oedema – Swelling from excessive accumulation of fluid in the body's tissues

Opacity – An opaque or non-transparent area appearing light or white on a radiograph (*plural:* **opacities**) – *also see* **radiopaque**

Organogenesis – The formation and development of organs

Ossification – The process of bone formation

PACS – *See* **picture archiving and communication system**

Parenchyma – The functional parts of an organ in the body. This is in contrast to the stroma, which refers to the structural tissue of organs, namely, the connective tissues

Pedicle – The segment of bone between the transverse process and vertebral body, forming part of the vertebral arch of each vertebra

Percutaneous – Passed, done or effected through the skin

Perforation – A hole or break in the containing walls or membranes of an organ or structure of the body

Periphery – The outermost boundary of an area; the surface of an object

Peristalsis – The coordinated wavelike contraction of smooth muscle that forces food through the digestive tract

Peritoneal cavity – The interior of the peritoneum, the lining of the abdominal cavity

Peritoneal dialysis – An alternative to haemodialysis used to manage patients with severe chronic kidney disease. Fluid is drained in and out of the peritoneal cavity on a regular basis to remove waste products from the blood by using the peritoneal membrane in the abdomen as a natural filter

Peritonitis – Inflammation of the peritoneum

Phlebolith – A small, rounded, calcification within a vein, commonly seen in the pelvis

Picture archiving and communication system (PACS) – A computer-based digital radiograph storage system for storing X-ray images, thereby eliminating the need for film

Pleural effusion – A condition that results from fluid accumulating in the pleural cavity in the chest

Pneumobilia – Also known as aerobilia is accumulation of gas in the biliary tree

Pneumonia – An inflammatory condition of the lung caused by bacterial or viral infection

Pneumoperitoneum – Gas in the peritoneal cavity

Pneumoretroperitoneum – Gas in the retroperitoneal space

Portal vein – A short vein formed by the confluence of the splenic and superior mesenteric veins, draining blood from the bowel and spleen into the liver

Post-operative – After surgery

Proximal – Situated close to the centre, median line, or point of attachment or origin

Pseudopolyps – An 'island' of preserved colonic mucosa, surrounded by ulcerated mucosa, such that it resembles a polyp

Pyeloplasty – Surgical reconstruction of the renal pelvis to correct an obstruction

Radiograph – An X-ray image

Radiolucent – Allowing the passage of X-rays. Radiolucent structures appear dark or near black on a conventional radiograph

Radiopaque – Obstructing the passage of X-rays. Radiopaque structures appear light or white on a conventional radiograph

Radiosensitive – Sensitive to the effects of radiation

Renal – Relating to the kidney

Renal tubular acidosis – A syndrome characterised by decreased ability of the kidneys to acidify urine, and by low plasma bicarbonate and high plasma chloride concentrations, often with hypokalemia

Retroperitoneum – The retroperitoneal space; the space between the peritoneum and the posterior abdominal wall (*adjective:* **retroperitoneal**)

Rigler's sign – Also known as the 'double-wall sign'; the radiographic appearance of gas present on both sides of the bowel wall as seen in pneumoperitoneum

Rigler's triad – Three radiographic findings seen in gallstone ileus consisting of pneumobilia, small bowel obstruction and gallstone

Rugae (of the stomach) – The large ridges or folds seen in the mucous membrane of the stomach

Sclerosis (of bone) – Abnormal area of increased density within the bone (*adjective:* **sclerotic**)

Sentinel loop – A localised distended loop of small bowel seen on an abdominal radiograph; caused by a localised ileus close to an intra-abdominal inflammatory process such as pancreatitis

Sphincter of Oddi – A muscular valve that controls the flow of digestive juices (bile and pancreatic juices) through the ampulla of Vater into the second part of the duodenum

Sphincterotomy – Incision or division of a sphincter muscle

Splenomegaly – Enlargement of the spleen

Staghorn calculus – A large calculus occurring in the renal pelvis, with branches extending into the calyces

Strangulation (of the bowel) – Constriction of a segment of bowel so as to cut off the flow of blood; a potential complication of bowel herniation

Stricture – An abnormal narrowing or stenosis of a duct or passage, usually caused by inflammation, external pressure or scarring

Superior – Higher in place or position, the opposite of inferior

Supine – Lying on the back with face upward

Suprapubic – Pertaining to a location above the pubic symphysis

Syndesmophyte – A bony growth attached to a ligament. It is found between adjacent vertebrae in ankylosing spondylitis

Taenia coli – Three thickened bands formed by the longitudinal fibres in the tunica muscularis of the large intestine, extending from the root of the appendix to the rectum

Teratogenesis – The production of congenital anomalies or defects in the developing embryo

Thumbprinting – The radiographic appearance of 'thumb-shaped' projections into the bowel lumen caused by severe thickening of the haustral folds of the colon

Tissue – An aggregation of similarly specialized cells which together perform certain special functions

Tortuous – Having many twists and turns

Toxic megacolon – Acute dilation of the colon; a serious complication of ulcerative colitis that may be life threatening

Tumour – An abnormal swelling or mass of tissue

Ulcerative colitis – A type of inflammatory bowel disease that only affects the large intestine (colon) and rectum

Ultrasound – A diagnostic medical imaging technique using ultrasound waves to visualise internal body structures

Undifferentiated – Refers to a group of diagnoses in which there is no differentiation from the underlying pathoanatomical diagnosis

Urological – Relating to the medical specialty concerned with the urinary system in both males and females, and the genital organs in the male

Uropathy – A disorder involving the urinary tract

Uterine fibroid (leiomyoma) – A benign smooth muscle tumour arising from the uterine myometrium

Valvulae conniventes – The mucosal folds of the small intestine. They have a characteristic appearance on an abdominal radiograph (*see page 30*)

Volvulus – Abnormal twisting of the bowel on its mesentery causing obstruction

Index